Jamaican Gold

To: Olayinka
Best wishes and enjoy reading
Wilma Charlton
Olympian 64, 68, 72
August 6, 2012
Rachael Irving

Jamaican Gold

Jamaican Sprinters

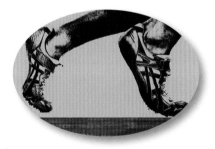

EDITED BY **RACHAEL IRVING** AND **VILMA CHARLTON**

UNIVERSITY OF THE WEST INDIES PRESS

Jamaica • Barbados • Trinidad and Tobago

University of the West Indies Press
7A Gibraltar Hall Road   Mona
Kingston 7   Jamaica
www.uwipress.com

ISBN 978-976-640-234-1

A catalogue record of this book is available from the National Library of Jamaica.

Cover photograph © Patrik Giardino/CORBIS

Book and cover design by Robert Harris.

Set in Fairfield LH Light 11/15

Printed in China by Regent Publishing Services

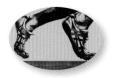

Contents

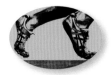

Foreword

For over five decades, a situation accelerated by the tremendous successes of our athletes at the Beijing Olympic Games, people all over the world have been fascinated by or remain in disbelief at the achievements of Jamaican athletes at the world level.

Dr Rachael Irving, researcher at the University of the West Indies, and Vilma Charlton, an Olympian, have for some time been soliciting the views of a wide cross-section of athletes and have put together a most informative approach as seen by various authors. I have, on my own, evaluated each presentation and can only conclude that the discussions on our athletes' successes will continue well beyond this publication.

The authors must be congratulated for their perseverance and it is my sincere hope that they will pursue every new approach that may be placed before them and what could become volume 2 of their work.

NEVILLE "TEDDY" McCOOK

Past President, Jamaica Amateur Athletic Association (JAAA)
President, North America, Central America and Caribbean
  Athletic Association (NACAC)
Council Member, International Association of Athletics
  Federations (IAAF)

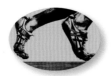

Acknowledgements

riting a book requires the combined effort of a team. To all the authors and editors, we say thanks in a big way.

Special thanks to Yannis Pitsiladis and the research team from the University of Glasgow, Scotland, who came up with the idea of studying the genetics of Jamaican elite athletes. Many thanks to Jamaica Amateur Athletic Association (JAAA), Jamaica Olympic Association (JOA), Olympians Association of Jamaica (OAJ), United States Olympic Committee (USOC) and USA Track and Field (USATF). A special handshake goes out to the very knowledgeable coach Stephen Francis and the Maximizing Velocity and Power (MVP) Track Club. Stephen constantly argues that Jamaicans must be involved in the documentation and research of their elite athletes. Thanks, Stephen, you are a true Jamaican. We will always remember Herb McKenley for the guidance he gave. Before we conceptualized this book, at the beginning of our study of Jamaican athletes, Herb made a profound statement: "Science without history is useless." You are not here to read this tribute; nevertheless, thanks, Mr McKenley. Vilma and I have combined science and history in writing this book. To Leslie and Pamela Laing, 1948 Olympians: What a team you make! Your thoughts and instructions as we viewed Jamaica from the penthouse on Kingston's waterfront remain invaluable. Peter Williams of Rosehall Developments Limited is a visionary in regard to the development of tourism in Jamaica. Thanks, Peter, for your remarkable advocacy for the combination of scientific research, sports and tourism. You spoke about writing and we have heeded your advice. Janet Silvera of Hospitality Jamaica convinced us that we had a story to tell the world. Thanks, Janet, we know now that the world has been waiting patiently to read *Jamaican Gold*.

Thanks to the students from G.C. Foster College, who were responsible for providing us with the majority of the control samples for the speed gene (actinin 3) analysis in Jamaicans. Thanks to the managers, coaches and elite athletes who gave us permission to use valuable images. We greatly appreciate the enormous support given to us by the *Jamaica Observer* in allowing us to use the fantastic images captured at the Beijing Olympics, and the twelfth IAAF World Championships in Athletics, Berlin, and elsewhere, by their chief photographer Brian Cummings. Special thanks to Olympian Rupert Hoilett for his invaluable support on the ground. Thanks to Charlie Fuller, who confirmed all our statistics on the individual athletes' performances, and Dr Paul Auden, who guided us in some of the history about our ancestors.

To our many colleagues and friends who supported us in ensuring that the quality of this book is remarkable, we are grateful. We could not have done it without your support.

We say thanks to our children, Bridgette and Kristie, who also gave good advice and guidance.

Finally to God, we give our accolades. Summing it all up: "I have considered the days of old, the years of ancient times" (Psalms 77:5), and "The lines are fallen unto me in pleasant places; yea, I have a goodly heritage" (Psalms 16:6).

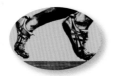

Introduction

The sparkle started at the 1948 Olympics in London, when the "gentle giant", Arthur Wint, won Jamaica's first gold medal in the 400 metres. Four years later at the 1952 Olympics in Helsinki, the excitement was palpable when the quartet of Leslie Laing, Arthur Wint, Herb McKenley and George Rhoden edged out the favourite US team in the 4 × 400-metre relay by a tenth of a second to set a new world record of 3:03.9 seconds. Jamaica was not, then, an independent nation but a colony of Britain. Jamaica became independent in 1962, and its presence at the Olympics under the black, green and gold flag has been remarkable. The chronicle of sustained medal achievement is truly phenomenal. In 1968, Lennox Miller won silver in the 100 metres at the Olympics in Mexico City. By 1976, his teammate Donald O'Reilly Quarrie had joined him in the rank of medal winners, winning gold in the 200 metres and silver in the 100 metres. Merlene Ottey took the Jamaican women near enough to the pinnacle in 1980 when she won a bronze in the 200 metres at the Moscow Olympics. Other women were to follow by taking us nearer with silver medals; however, it was the unassuming Deon Hemmings who broke the trend, to become the first Jamaican woman to win an Olympic gold. By 2004 in Athens, Veronica Campbell-Brown was crying as she collected gold for the 200 metres. The euphoria was felt all over the world in August 2008 as Jamaican sprinters collected seven out of twelve available medals in the men's and women's 100- and 200-metre events at the Beijing Olympics. Jamaicans not only collected medals but set three world records and an Olympic record. Usain Bolt's "To the World" signal at the Bird's Nest, Beijing's Olympic stadium, left an indelible mark.

Jamaica's performance at the 2009 IAAF World Championships in Berlin reinforced the title and image of "Sprint Capital of the World". Europeans with diverse accents labelled themselves Jamaicans-of-Berlin.

By the end of the games, Jamaica had amassed thirteen medals, which included seven gold, four silver and two bronze. Although the United States had surpassed the Jamaicans in terms of total medal count, Jamaicans dominated in sprint events. Alison Felix, as she defeated Veronica Campbell-Brown of Jamaica in the 200-metre final, was able to clip Jamaica's sweep of the 100- and 200-metre sprints. Shelly-Ann Fraser's indelible smile as she won the 100 metres in a time of 10.73 seconds, with Kerron Stewart in close second with a time of

10.75 seconds, and Melaine Walker's championship record of 52.42 seconds in the 400-metre hurdles placed the world at Jamaica's feet.

Why is Jamaica as a small nation so highly represented on the medal podium in the international sprint events? The world is seeking answers. Jamaica, a small nation with less than three million people, is classified as a developing country with limited resources, yet the successes of Jamaican athletes have been sustained over decades.

The phenomenal success of Jamaicans in sprint events is bewildering to many. Thus, the idea for this book grew out of the many questions, myths and hypotheses surrounding "Brand Jamaica" athletics. The editors and authors have sought to provide an overview of available data on the historical profiles, genetics, biomechanics, psychological factors, physical conditioning and the "speed agent" (yam) that might be linked to Jamaican sprinting prowess. To eliminate bias, two European authors have compared notes with Jamaicans on athletic prowess in Caucasians and people of African descent. Anti-doping and protection strategies are topical and relevant to Jamaica's athletic programmes; therefore, these areas are covered in the book. Included, too, are the human stories that make Jamaica's athletics seem almost mythical. This book, a Jamaica-storied, scientific history, is divided into sections, where information can be analysed as a unit or separately, depending on your preference. The separation of different topics is to facilitate those who just want to read lightly as well as others who are more scientifically inclined and want to delve deeply into data. Exploring athletics in Jamaica in sections adds a deeper dimension to the story surrounding Jamaica, the sprint capital of the world.

The first section truly distinguishes this book: it provides historical evidence supported by scientific data and proposed compensatory mechanisms that have favourable relationships with sprinting. This section is remarkable because of the conflicting views on the interpretation of the scientific data by the Jamaican and European authors. Strength, flexibility, power evaluation and injury management in athletic prowess are examined. Coaches will benefit from the chapter on physical therapy, which characterizes injury management and different approaches to treatment of sports injuries. The value and importance of natural tubers grown in Jamaica to nutrition and medicine are not well elucidated in worldwide literature. A thorough outline of the different yams found in different regions of the world and their various usages is aptly done by Helen Asemota, an African professor and consultant to the Food and Agricultural Organization of the United Nations who has made Jamaica her home.

The human triumph and lives of some trailblazers are highlighted in section 2. The emergence of Jamaica as a dominant force in sprinting is aptly illustrated by Jimmy Carnegie as he writes about its seven decades of participation in the Olympics. The almost mythical life of the oldest living Jamaican Olympian is explored, as is the life of the only person in 112 years of competition who ever set three world records in track and field at a single Olympics and who went on, a year later in Berlin, to reset two of those three world records. In this section lies the story of the hurdler who set an Olympic record in Beijing and then went on to set a championship record in the 400-metre hurdles at the twelfth IAAF World Championships in Athletics in Berlin.

Section 3 is a photographic essay presenting images of Jamaica's mastery in sprinting.

We cannot have Jamaican athletics without humour. Section 4 speaks to the cultural norms that make us unique. Laugh as renowned psychiatrist, sports psychology specialist and percussionist Dr Aggrey Irons presents "Run for Your Life", a portrayal of Jamaicans' fascination with running. In this section, too, is the history of Jamaica's Boys' and Girls' Championships. Bobby Fray traces one hundred years of boys' and, later, girls' running. This annual championship meet provides the psychological tools that hone sprinting ability.

Section 5 provides a detailed analysis of current anti-doping practices and recommends measures that must be implemented to protect elite athletes and expose cheaters in this era of gene hacking, doping and supplement label omission.

The authors may not provide all the answers, but they provide historical, scientific and cultural information that will help guide impartial analysis of the sprinting prowess of Jamaican athletes. The writers have considered the controversies associated with athletics in Jamaica as well. After reading *Jamaican Gold*, readers, we hope, will understand some of the factors that make Jamaican athletes truly remarkable. The authors are sure that the readers will find here a wealth of information.

SECTION 1

The Science of Jamaica's Sprinting Ability

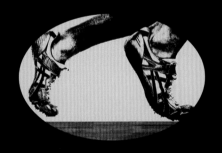

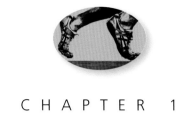

Why Jamaica Rules in Sprinting

University Research Explores the Reasons

R A C H A E L   I R V I N G   A N D   V I L M A   C H A R L T O N

Jamaica's prowess at the twenty-ninth Olympiad in Beijing, China, and twelfth IAAF World Championships in Berlin, Germany, has left many wondering how such a tiny nation of approximately 2.7 million people can outrun nations such as the United States and Britain, whose athletes previously dominated in the sprint events.

Jamaica's sprinting evolution can be traced back to 1952, when the quartet of Herb McKenley, George Rhoden, Arthur Wint and Leslie Laing set the stadium in Helsinki on fire by breaking the world record in the 4×400-metre relay. The country's performance nearly reached its zenith at the twenty-ninth Olympiad. The country's performance at the twelfth IAAF World Championships in Athletics in Berlin was mind-boggling and elicited responses of shock and disbelief. In a sport marred by illegal steroid use and recent gene doping, Jamaica's record-breaking haul of six gold, three silver and two bronze medals in Beijing and seven gold,

four silver and two bronze medals in Berlin has been met with suspicion and many questions.

Why are Jamaicans excelling in sprint events at the international level? The University of Glasgow in Scotland and the University of the West Indies (UWI) in the Caribbean are hoping to give definitive answers as to the cause of this phenomenon. Both universities have embarked on a collaborative study to examine the role of genetics, environment and physical education and training in Jamaica's athletic success.

Initial results from work done over a two-year period suggest a genetic predisposition in Jamaicans. The researchers have discovered that DNA analyses carried out on 120 Jamaican Olympians, with controls consisting of 200 ordinary Jamaicans, showed that 75 per cent of the Olympians have the strong 577RR variant of the alpha actinin 3 (ACTN3) gene, a gene which established research has proved is associated with fast-twitch muscle fibres that allow for high velocity or power

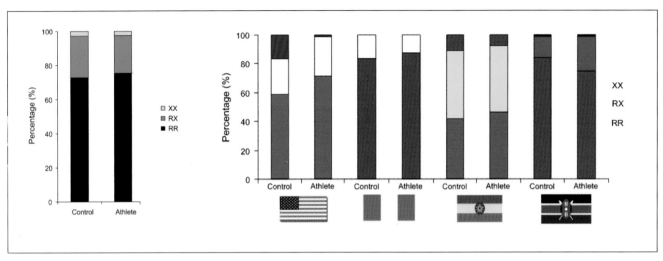

FIGURE 1.1 ACTN3 (the sprint gene) profiles: Jamaica vs United States, Nigeria, Ethiopia and Kenya.

sprinting. The actinin 3 gene is a performance-related gene, and one must have the strong form 577RR (homozygous) or the weaker form 577RX (heterozygous) to produce the protein alpha actinin 3 that is associated with power sprinting.

Most persons of West African ancestry have the 577RR or 577RX variant. Only about 1 per cent of West Africans have the 577XX or null variant, which does not produce the sprint protein. In Jamaica, the null form is found in approximately 2 per cent of the population, while this cohort is 4 per cent in the United States (Irving et al. 2009), absent in Nigerians, 11 per cent in Ethiopians and 1 per cent in Kenyans (Yang et al. 2007).

It is ironic that 75 per cent of the ordinary Jamaicans tested have the 577RR variant (Scott et al. 2010). Where does that leave us? Does this say that any Jamaican can be a Usain Bolt or Asafa Powell? Yes and no, and please do not be confused by the answer. Jamaicans are genetically predisposed to be sprinters, because of their shared ancestry with West Africans;

however, the gene has to be switched on or off by environmental factors and physical conditioning.

Examining the genetic predisposition to diabetes, one can relate prevalence to environment and draw an analogy to genetic predisposition to sprinting and a nurturing environment in Jamaican athletes. One might have a family history of diabetes but the disease may not be manifested if one eats correctly and exercises. Many families with diabetes have been studied, and we will speak of a classical family X. Mr X's mother had diabetes, and his four sisters were overweight and all had diabetes before age thirty-five years. Mr X's six daughters and one son had diabetes, but Mr X never developed diabetes because he walked ten miles per day, was a vegetarian and remained lean all his life. The very same phenomenon is seen in athletes. The environment affects the sprint gene, actinin 3, in a positive or negative way. So, if the environment is not conductive, you may have the gene but fail to perform well on the track.

The DNA samples of the Jamaicans were analysed

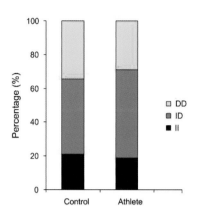

FIGURE 1.2 The variants in Jamaicans of the ACE gene implicated in oxygen flow in the body.

for another performance-related gene, the angiotensin-converting enzyme (ACE), gene. This gene is involved in the regulation of blood volume, blood flow and oxygen delivery. The DD and DI variants of the ACE gene in our elite athletes account for 52 per cent and 29 per cent and in ordinary Jamaicans account for 47 per cent and 36 per cent, which are statistically similar. It is ironic that the II variant of the ACE gene that is negatively associated with sprinting was found in less than 20 per cent of the Jamaican population (Olympians and controls).

It cannot be said that the ACE gene, however, is helping the sprinters to perform because the profile of this gene is the same in elite runners as well as non-performing Jamaicans. The DD and DI variants of the ACE gene that

are positively associated with sprinting (Nazarov et al. 2001) are also associated with increased prevalence of diabetes, hypertension and cardiovascular disease (Esteghamati et al. 2007). Jamaica has a point prevalence of 17.5 per cent diabetes in persons older than fifteen years (Ragoorbirsingh et al. 1995).

In addition to carrying out DNA analyses on Jamaicans who participated in the 1948 Olympics right through to those who participated in the twenty-ninth Olympiad, tests were also conducted on one hundred national athletes (those who participated locally and in the Caribbean) and three hundred persons from the Cockpit Country and Trelawny region of Jamaica. The latter cohort was included because many Olympians either have emerged from that area or have links there. Interestingly, the profile of the persons from the Cockpit Country is similar to that of the Olympians.

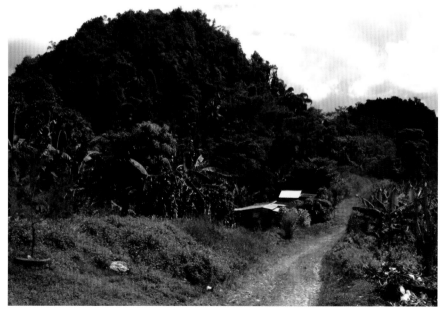

PLATE 1.1 Many Jamaican Olympians have their roots in the Cockpit Country area of Trelawny, in western Jamaica. (Photograph by Martin Mordecai.)

The persons from the Cockpit Country have a high frequency of 577RR, the ACTN3 variant associated with elite sprinting. Having the 577RR variant of the actinin 3 gene does not explain why Jamaicans dominate in international sprint events. There must be something driving this gene and/or other genes to perform to the full potential. When something drives a gene or switches it on or off, it is termed "gene environmental effect". We postulate that there are special minerals in the Cockpit Country, akin to bauxites, that the plants uptake and Jamaicans eat in yam and other tubers. Many Olympians, such as Usain Bolt, Veronica Campbell-Brown, Donovan Bailey and Deon Hemmings, come from that region. Even more of the parents of Olympians are from the Cockpit Country.

Muscular properties are subjected to inherited influences. Muscle fibres numbers are determined by the second trimester of pregnancy. So even before birth our Olympians are influenced by their environment.

The phenomenon seen in the Cockpit Country region of Jamaica could be similar to the one found in the Rift Valley region of Kenya, which has proved to be a fertile area for the development of world-beating athletes in long-distance events.

Physical education has come a long way in Jamaica and we are fortunate to have a programme in our schools and events like Boys' and Girls' Athletic Championships for schools. We are also fortunate to have the G.C. Foster College, which trains teachers and coaches so that our schools have qualified persons to help with the teaching and training of the athletes.

The Jamaican programme has had an impact on athletics internationally. The IAAF president, Lamine Diack, has even praised it, because Jamaica definitely has something that is working.

References

Esteghamati, A., A.R. Nikzamir, R. Rashidi and M. Zahraei. 2007. The relationship between the insertion/deletion polymorphism of the ACE gene and hypertension in Iranian patients with type 2 diabetes. *Nephrology Dialysis Transplantation* 22 (9): 2549–53.

Irving, R., R. Scott, L. Irwin, E. Morrison, V. Charlton, A. Austin, S. Headley, F. Kolkhorst and Y. Pitsiladis. 2009. The ACTN3 R577X polymorphism in elite Jamaican and USA sprinters. *Medicine and Science in Sports and Exercise* 41 (5): 1067.

Nazarov, I.B., D.R. Woods, H.E. Montgomery, O.V. Shneider, V.I. Kazakov, N.V. Tomilin and V.A. Rogozkin. 2001. The angiotensin converting enzyme I/D polymorphism in Russian athletes. *European Journal of Human Genetics* 9:797–801.

Ragoorbirsingh D., G. Lewis-Fuller and E.Y. Morrison. 1995. The Jamaican diabetes survey. A protocol for the Caribbean. *Diabetes Care* 18 (9): 1277–79.

Scott, R., R. Irving, L. Irwin, M. Morrison, V. Charlton, K. Austin, D. Tladi, A. Headley, F. Kolkhorst, N. Yang, K. North and Y.P. Pitsiladis. 2010. ACTN3 and ACE genotypes in elite Jamaican and US sprinters. *Medicine and Science in Sports and Exercise* 42 (1): 107–15.

Yang, N., DaG. MacArthur, B. Wolde, V. Onywera, K. Boit, S.Y. Lau, R.H. Wilson, R.A. Scott, Y.P. Pitsiladis and K. North. 2007. The ACTN3 R577X polymorphism in East and West African athletes. *Medicine and Science in Sports and Exercise* 39 (11): 1985–88.

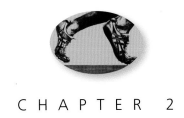

CHAPTER 2

Charting the Ancestry of Elite Jamaican and US Sprinters

RACHAEL IRVING

The transatlantic slave trade lasted over three centuries and was instrumental in moving millions of people from Africa to the Americas. The first set of slave labourers arrived in the Americas in the early sixteenth century (Thomas 1997). The transatlantic slave trade transported an estimated 11 million people from Africa, with about one third from West Africa, to Europe and the Americas (Torres et al. 2007). The mitochondrial DNA (mtDNA) genome of the descendants of these transported people has retained an imprint of the process. A database of thousands of MtDNAs, including MtDNA sequences from Africa, are publicly available and mitochondrial lineages of West African ancestry in the Caribbean and North America have been identified through genomic analyses (Salas et al. 2005).

Mitochondrial DNA has been linked to physical performance and trainability (Rivera et al. 1998), but more

important is that mitochondrial DNA markers or haplogroups can be used in the creation of detailed phylogenies or biogeography charts to explore the matrilineal relatedness of people. Mitochondrial haplogroup distributions are sensitive to population history and some studies have looked at haplogroup distributions in the Caribbean (Parra et al. 1998; Torres et al. 2007). The few studies to date that have included Jamaica have suggested a predominately West African ancestry with few genetic inroads by Europeans and Asians (Dunn 1977; Torres et al. 2007). Similar studies done on various African-American groups in the United States have indicated a variable admixture, with the rates of European lineages increasing away from former slave states and northern and western cities (McLean et al. 2003; Parra et al. 1998).

There is growing interest in the genetic trace of the ancestry of Caribbean and US elite sprinters because

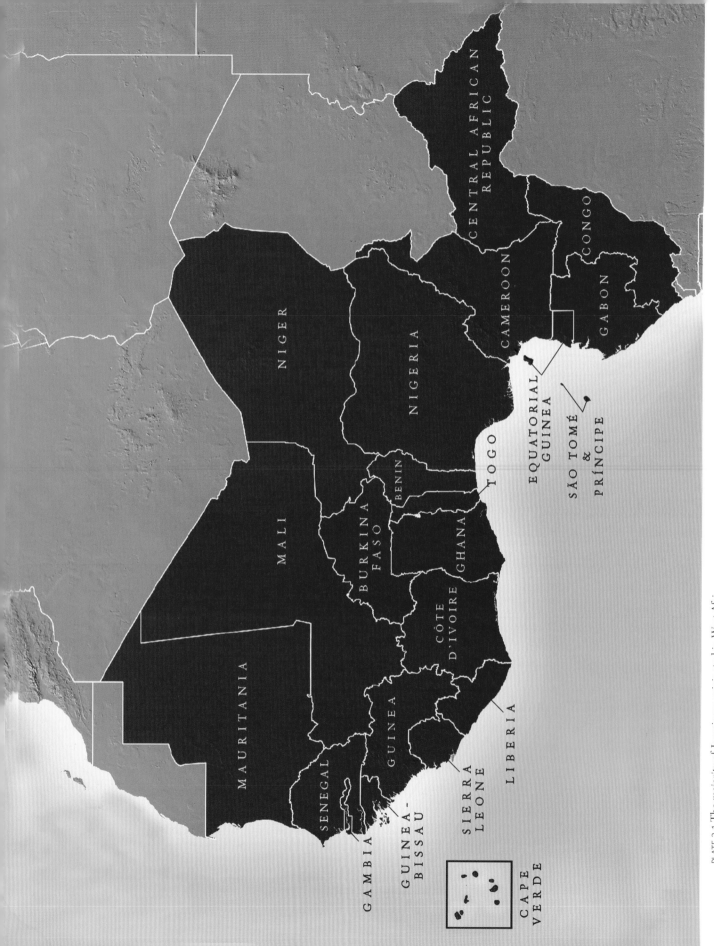

PLATE 2.1 The majority of Jamaicans originated in West Africa.

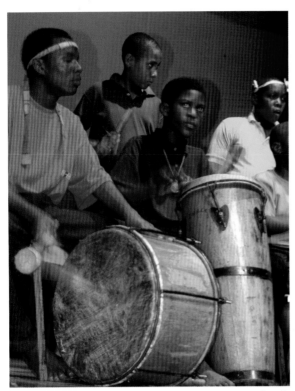

PLATE 2.2 Jamaican children are exposed to important cultural elements of their African heritage through the Jamaica Cultural Development Corporation's Annual Festival of Arts. (Jamaica Information Service photograph.)

of the disproportionate success of these athletes in international events. Historical records indicate that the current male record-holders for the short distances (100 to 400 metres) and hurdles and the late Florence "Flo-Jo" Griffith-Joyner, female world record holder for the 100- and 200-metre sprints, descended from West Africa. While MtDNA haplogroup distributions in the Caribbean and United States are well researched (Martinez-Cruzado et al. 2001; Martinez-Cruzado et al. 2005; Salas et al. 2005; Torres et al. 2007), the lineage trace of elite Jamaican and US sprinters has never been untaken before this study.

Researchers from the University of the West Indies, the University of Glasgow and Florida State University collected samples from 107 and 119 elite Jamaican and US athletes(JA_A and USA_A) respectively. Samples were also collected from 293 Jamaicans and 1,148 African Americans (JA_C and USA_C) who have not participated in sports at the national level. The first hyperviable region (HVR-1) of MtDNA was sequenced for each participant and samples were haplogrouped according to the comprehensive full mitochondrial DNA genome phylogenetic tree (van-Oven and Kayser 2009). The haplotypic distribution for the Jamaican and African-American cohorts was evaluated.

The majority of Jamaican athletes (98 per cent) possessed L1b, L2b, L2c, L2d, L3b and L3d haplogroups characteristic of West Africa and L1c and L3e characteristic of West-Central Africa (Salas et al. 2005). Two Jamaican athletes were characterized as having haplogroups typical of non-sub-Saharan Africa. The US athletes had mainly haplogroups L1b, L2b, L2c, L2d L3b, L3d, L1c and L3e, suggestive of West and West-Central African ancestry, and the L4/L7 haplogroup not found in Jamaican athletes was present in the US sprinters (table 2.1). The L4/L7 haplogroup is associated with East Africa and West Eurasia. Haplogroup L4 is present at high frequencies in Tanzanian click-speaking populations (Tishkoff et al. 2007). The African-American sprinters had more non-L/U6 or a greater percentage of European admixture than the Jamaican sprinters (10 per cent versus 2 per cent). Twenty-one of the US athletes were of European ancestry (non-L/U6) and three of Asian ancestry.

The athletes from Jamaica and their controls had similar haplogroup distributions predicative of West and West-Central African origin, and although the controls had more admixture with Eurasia and Asia, it was not

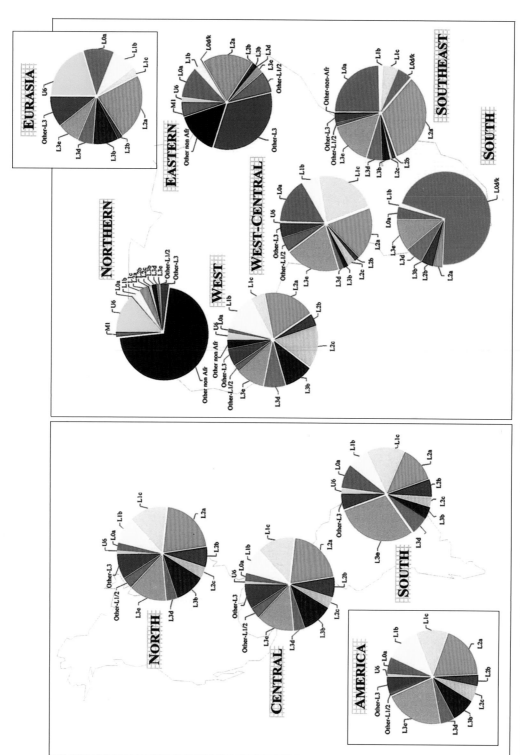

FIGURE 2.1 Frequency profiles of the major haplogroups in Africa and haplogroups of recent African ancestry in the Americas and Eurasia (Salas et al. 2004).

significant. The study proved that mitochondrial haplogroup distributions in elite Jamaican sprinters and ordinary Jamaicans (controls) are similar and are primarily derived from the same source populations in West and West-Central Africa. The results indicate that there is no population isolation or stratification along lines of sprint performance.

The haplogroup diversity between the African Americans who participated in national-level sports and those who did not (controls) was significant. Ninety-four of the controls had the non-L/U6 haplogroup and nine the U6 haplogroup. No African-American athlete had the U6 haplogroup. The U6 is the autochthonous haplogroup of North Africa (Salas et al. 2005). Mitochondrial lineage might therefore have an impact on performance in African Americans, as seen in Japanese and Finnish athletes (Niemi et al. 2005; Mikami et al. 2010).

Mitochondrial haplogroups and biogeography frequency charts are based on specific population histories (Alves-Silva et al. 2000; Bandelt et al. 2001; Salas et al. 2004). This lineage research indicates that Jamaican and African-American sprinters are mainly of West or West-Central African ancestry. The greater mitochondrial diversity in African-American sprinters as compared to the Jamaican sprinters indicates that isolation, differences in number and source of Africans imported, and colonization history may impact population genetics and the performance of US sprinters.

Table 2.1 Mitochondrial Lineages of Elite Jamaican and US Sprinters and Their Respective Controls

Haplogroups	JA_A (107)	JA_C (293)	USA_A (119)	USA_C (1148)
L0a	7	13	2	41
L1b	14	33	13	105
L1c	13	18	8	126
L2a	23	86	15	216
L2b	3	15	8	55
L2c	6	13	7	57
L3b	5	19	3	90
L3d	3	13	7	75
L3e	21	39	16	194
L3f	5	20	11	55
L4/L7	0	0	1	4
L5	1	1	0	0
Non-L/U6	2	5	25	94
Other L0'1'2	3	10	3	12
Other L3	1	6	0	15
U6	0	2	0	9

References

Alves-Silva, J., M. Santos, P. Guimarães, A.C. Ferreira, H-J. Bandelt, S.D. Pena and V.F. Prado. 2000. The ancestry of Brazilian mtDNA lineages. *American Journal of Human Genetics* 67:444–61.

Bandelt, H-J., J. Alves-Silva, P. Guimarães, M. Santos, M. Brehm, L. Pereira, A. Coppa, J.M. Larruga, C. Rengo, R. Scozzari, A. Torroni, M.J. Prata, A. Amorim, V.F. Prado and S.D.J. Pena. 2001. Phylogeography of the human mitochondrial L3e: A snapshot of African prehistory and Atlantic slave trade. *Annals of Human Genetics* 65:549–63.

Dunn, R. 1977. A tale of two plantations: Slave life at Mesopotamia in Jamaica and Mount airy in Virginia, 1799 to 1828. *William and Mary Quarterly* 34 (1): 32–65.

Martinez-Cruzado, J.C., G. Toro-Labrador, V. Ho-Fung, M.A. Estevez-Montero, A. Lobaina-Manzanet, D.A. Padovani-Claudio, H. Sanchez-Cruz, P. Ortiz-Bermudez and A. Sanchez-Crespo. 2001. Mitochondrial DNA analysis reveals substantial Native American ancestry in Puerto Rico. *Human Biology* 73:491–511.

Martinez-Cruzado, J.C., G. Toro-Labrador, J. Viera-Vera, M.Y. Rivera-Vega, J. Startek, M. Latorre-Esteves, A. Roman-Colon, R. Rivera-Torres, I.Y. Navarro-Millan, E. Gomez-Sanchez, H.Y. Caro-Gonzalez and P. Valencia-Rivera. 2005. Reconstructing the population history of Puerto Rico by means of mtDNA phylogeographic analysis. *American Journal of Physical Anthropology* 128 (1): 131–55.

McLean D.C., Jr., I. Spruill, S. Gevao, E.Y. Morrison, O.S. Bernard, G. Argyropoulos and W.T. Garvey. 2003. Three novel mtDNA restriction site polymorphisms allow exploration of population affinities of African Americans. *Human Biology* 75 (2): 147–61.

Mikami, E., N. Fuku, H. Takahashi, N. Ohiwa, R.A. Scott, Y.P. Pitsiladis, M. Higuchi, T. Kawahara and M. Tanaka. 2010. Mitochondrial haplogroups associated with elite Japanese athlete status. *British Journal of Sports Medicine.* Online First: http://bjsm.bmj.com/content/early/2010/06/14/bjsm.2010.072371.

Niemi, A., and K. Majamaa. 2005. Mitochondrial DNA and ACTN3 genotypes in Finnish elite endurance and sprint athletes. *European Journal of Human Genetics* 13 (8): 965–69.

Parra, E.J., A. Marcini, J. Akey, J. Martinson, M.A. Batzer, R.

Cooper, T. Forrester, D.B. Allison, R. Deka, R.E. Ferrell and M.D. Shriver. 1998. Estimating African American admixture proportions by use of population-specific alleles. *American Journal of Human Genetics* 63:1839–51.

Rivera, M.A., B. Wolfarth, F.T. Dionne, M. Chagnon, J.A. Simoneau, M.R. Boulay, T.M. Song, L. Perusse, J. Gagnon, A.S. Leon, D.C. Rao, J.S. Skinner, J.H. Wilmore, J. Keul and C. Bouchard. 1998. Three mitochondrial DNA restriction polymorphisms in elite endurance athletes and sedentary controls. *Medicine and Science in Sports and Exercise* 30 (5): 687–90.

Salas, A., M. Richards, T. De la Fé, M-V. Lareu, B. Sobrino, P. Sánchez-Diz, V. Macaulay and A. Carracedo. 2002. The making of the African mtDNA landscape. *American Journal of Human Genetics* 71:1082–111.

Salas, A., M. Richards, M-V. Lareu, R. Scozzari, A. Coppa, A. Torroni, V. Macaulay and A. Carracedo. 2004. The African diaspora: Mitochondrial DNA and the Atlantic slave trade. *American Journal of Human Genetics* 74:454–65.

Salas, A., M. Richards, A. Carracedo and V. Macaulay. 2005. Charting the ancestry of African Americans. *American Journal of Human Genetics* 77:676–80.

Thomas, H. 1997. *The slave trade: The story of the Atlantic slave trade, 1440–1870.* New York: Simon and Schuster.

Tishkoff, S.A., M.K. Gonder, B. Henn, H. Mortensen, A. Knight, C. Gignoux, N. Fernandopulle, G. Lema, T.B. Nyambo, U. Ramakrishnan, F.A. Reed and J. Mountain. 2007. History of click-speaking populations of Africa inferred from mtDNA and Y chromosome genetic variation. *Molecular Biology and Evolution* 24 (10): 2180–95.

Toress, B.J., R.A. Kittles and A.C. Stone. 2007. Mitochondrial and Y chromosome diversity in the English-speaking Caribbean. *Annals of Human Genetics* 71:1–9.

van Oven, M., and M. Kayser. 2009. Updated comprehensive phylogenetic tree of global human mitochondrial DNA variation. *Human Mutation* 30 (2): E386–E394.

CHAPTER 3

Some Biomedical Mechanisms in Athletic Prowess

ERROL MORRISON AND PATRICK COOPER

For several decades the disproportionate success of individuals of African descent in a wide range of athletic activities has been the subject of intense speculation and debate. Today, despite being a mere 12 per cent of the American population, African Americans constitute a clear majority of that country's greatest athletes. Moreover, the disproportionate success in the area of sports, by the largely Afrocentric populations in the tiny islands of the Caribbean, begs the questions "Why?" and "How?" We will argue that not only do athletes such as Herb McKenley, Merlene Ottey, Asafa Powell, Michael Jordan, Carl Lewis, Pele, Tiger Woods, Muha-mmad Ali, Brian Lara and Garfield Sobers rank among the greatest performers of all time in their respective athletic activities, that they are athletes of tremendous raw physical ability and that they are of West African-related origin.

Hypothesis

We contend that there is substantial, documented evidence that the success of individuals of West African descent in athletic activities involving speed and power is based on biomechanical and biochemical differences between themselves and white and Asian athletes (Ama et al. 1990) and biochemical differences between themselves and all other Africans (Carlson 1984). Blacks from other parts of the African continent, led by the Kenyans, are now the greatest distance runners in the world. While those other Africans share some athletically advantageous biomechanisms with their West African cousins, it appears that they are similar to Europeans and all other racial and ethnic groups in fast-twitch/slow-twitch muscle fibre proportion and are unlike West African and West African-descended groups, who have a higher percentage of fast-twitch muscle fibres and elevated activities in several related metabolic pathways.

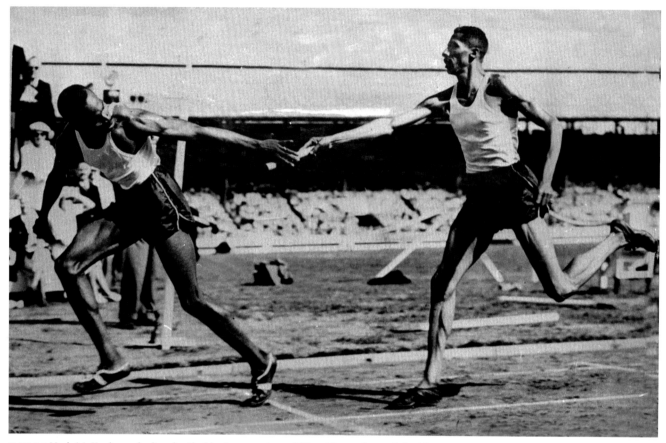

PLATE 3.1 Herb McKenley embodies the ideal body proportions of West African-descended athletes. Here he passes baton to George Rhoden in the gold-medal-winning performance in the 4 × 400-metre men's relay in the 1952 Helsinki Olympic Games. (*Gleaner* photograph.)

The African biomechanical advantages of lower subcutaneous fat, longer arms and legs, and narrower hips, which influence power-to-weight ratio and stride length, are well known and generally uncontroversial outcomes of human evolution in tropical climates. The essence of our hypothesis is our claim that the biochemical differences – essentially differences in glucose conversion rates – between West African and West African-descended populations and all other groups, including other black Africans, began but did not end with the sickling of the haemoglobin molecule. In the uniquely lethal West African malarial environment, individuals with the sickle-cell trait possessed a significant selective advantage. Although sickling is caused by a single amino acid substitution, valine for glutamic acid, encoding the sixth amino acid of the beta chain of the haemoglobin molecule, we will argue that the mutation triggered a series of physiological adjustments, which, incidentally, had favourable athletic consequences.

These adjustments, or compensatory mechanisms, include a higher percentage of fast-twitch muscle fibres, greater activity in the phosphagenic, glycolytic and lactate dehydrogenase metabolic pathways, and greater rate of ventilation, all of which have been scientifically tested and evaluated. These alterations affect the individual's process in storing and utilizing energy for skeletal muscle contraction and enhances the person's ability to build lean muscle mass.

Background

Plasmodium vivax, perhaps the oldest of the malaria types and once apparently ubiquitous throughout sub-Saharan Africa, has disappeared entirely in Africa, presumably because of a lack of hosts. The evidence for this assumption is the complete absence of Duffy antigen from the blood of more than 95 per cent of black Africans and those of African descent around the world, which makes them absolutely immune to that type of malarial parasite. The genetic characteristics known as the Duffy Antigenic System determine whether the *P. vivax* malaria parasite is able to penetrate the wall of the red blood cell. If either Duffy "a" or "b" type is present, penetration and infection can occur, but the "Duffy null" pattern prohibits invasion.

A new genetic defence, sickle-cell trait, and the biological adaptations it triggered – which apparently developed after the dispersion of the founders of the Bantu populations from their original West African homeland (between Cameroon and eastern Nigeria) – would not be possessed by the rest of Africa. The development of sickle-cell trait would have considerable medical and physiological consequences. Because these sickle-shaped cells are less hospitable to the malarial plasmodium than normal red blood cells, the debilitating effects of malarial infection are reduced in individuals who inherit this kind of red corpuscle from just one parent. But the cost of this biological protection, particularly before the advent of modern medicine, was high. Even today, in Africa, these individuals commonly die young. The inevitably higher rate of child mortality is further increased by the fact that those born entirely without the sickling gene are extremely vulnerable to lethal malarial infection.

While it is now indisputable that heterozygous individuals possess a selective advantage in areas of high malarial infection, the connection between sickle-cell trait and athletic ability or physical prowess was not immediately clear. In fact, since the sickle-cell gene reduces oxygen transportation in the circulatory system, the evidence apparently points in the opposite direction.

The hypothesis that the athletic prowess of people of West African origins is linked to their development of biological defences against falciparum malaria is not as new or as radical as it might seem. In 1954, British physician A.C. Allison first advanced the concept of sickling as an instance of natural selection in humans. Allison had spent several years in Africa drawing the blood of native people as part of an extensive colonial project to establish racial and tribal affinities. His familiarity with the findings of the malarial association allowed him to marshal the evidence required to support the hypothesis that carriers of the sickle-cell trait were immune to malaria.

It is also important to recognize that not all the athletic successes enjoyed by West Africans over Europeans and Asians are the result of mutations that took place in West Africa. Some, such as body proportions and low subcutaneous fat percentages, are shared, as stated earlier, with other Africans. The relatively shorter arms and legs and higher subcutaneous body fat of Europeans, Asians and all other non-African groups, which were adaptations to colder climates, are the result of mutations that occurred outside of Africa.

Somatotype and Genotype

The first indicator that individuals of West African descent had developed what would be described as "compensating mechanisms" as a response to the debilitating effects of sickle-cell trait came from an elaborate study of Olympic athletes from the 1968 Games in Mexico City. More than one thousand athletes, of both sexes, of every racial group and from all parts of the world, participated in the project, which was named the Program of Genetics and Human Biology. Unlike previous studies, which had been limited to the morphological basis of performance, the Mexico City study attempted to examine the possible genetic bases for body structure and sports performance. As a result, in addition to somatotyping, the Mexico City study collected and analysed a number of genetic and anthropological characteristics of the athletes.

Among the factors included were investigations of the sports histories of the families of the athletes; genetic traits of the athletes, especially those that might be correlated with sports ability; and those aspects of the athletes' physiques that represented the interaction of their genetic endowments with the environmental factors involved in training. The 1,265 athletes, representing 129 separate Olympic events, were grouped into four major racial categories: Caucasoid, Mongoloid, Mestizo (Indian plus Caucasoid) and Negroid. The classifications were based on identification and somatotype photographs, as well as physical characteristics including skin colour; general body shape; proportions of segments of the limbs; facial structure; form of eyes, lips and nose; and colour and texture of hair. Like the Tanner study of the athletes from the 1960 Olympic Games, the Mexico City survey confirmed the relationship between body type and athletic performance as well as the differences in body proportions between the Negroids and the other groups. Not only were the Negroids significantly narrower in hip breadth than the Caucasoids (slightly less so with the two other groups), but they were found to have longer arms and legs, and a shorter trunk, than the other groups. Despite these differences, the study concluded, "it would appear that the same somatotypes excel at the specified events regardless of race and that the functional requirements of the events demand similar somatotypes". However, the most interesting and important finding of the study was not produced by anthropometric measurements, but by tests to determine a possible association between athletic ability and single gene systems. Investigated were the ABO, MN and Rh red cell types; haptoglobin; glucose-6-phosphate dehydrogenase; and acid phosphatase. Although the study failed to link athletic ability to a single gene system, the authors expressed "surprise" that "a sizable number of Negroid Olympic athletes manifested the sickle-cell trait." The authors noted:

> In view of the importance of hemoglobin in the transport of oxygen to tissues, one might expect very slight differences in function or amount of hemoglobin to be reflected in athletic potential. Especially in the case of hemoglobin S (the sickle gene), one might suppose that the great oxygen demand, which accompanies certain athletic activities, might cause a certain amount of in vivo sickling of red cells even though this is not observed in heterozygotes under other conditions. Such persons might, therefore, be at a disadvantage, and even

a small disadvantage would be expected to prevent such persons attaining Olympic status. It was surprising to discover that this was not the case.

The surprising finding, that a shortage of haemoglobin had not adversely affected the athletic capabilities of black athletes, was magnified by the fact that the 1968 Olympics were staged at the high altitude of Mexico City. "One could imagine," the authors wrote, "that a greater oxygen deficit would be associated with this altitude and that persons heterozygous for haemoglobin S would be more likely to form sickle cells in vivo than at lower altitudes."

After pointing out that the genetic systems selected had been dictated primarily by the large number of athletes in the study, the researchers noted that when the study was planned, "the number of polymorphic protein and enzymes known was limited". However, they wrote, "This situation is changing rapidly, with new polymorphic enzyme systems being reported frequently." The systems, which with considerable foresight they found to be "of particular interest", were those "related to energy metabolism, where one might expect small differences in normal function to become important under the severe stress of athletic competition".

Eight years after the Mexico City report, an article in the *Journal of the National Medical Association*, the official organ of the African Medical Group, provided additional evidence that adjustments had been made in the energy-metabolizing systems of people of West African descent. The Mexico City study had expressed surprise that Negroid athletes with sickle-cell trait had been able to compete effectively at the highest levels, despite deficiencies in their oxygen transportation systems. This article, based on a massive study, would reveal, astonishingly, that not only was it individuals

with sickle-cell trait who had lower-than-average haemoglobin levels, but African Americans generally had significantly lower haemoglobin levels than their white counterparts. It would also raise, for the first time, the critical issue of how African Americans coped so well with this apparent biological handicap.

Conducted in ten states and in New York City, the study involved nearly thirty thousand individuals, divided into twenty-four age groups, from the first year through the ninth decade. To eliminate the possibility that the racial differences in haemoglobin levels were caused by socio-economic factors, the study included matched comparisons of blacks and whites with reported high levels of iron intake and higher incomes, and athletes of both races. Nonetheless, the results clearly indicated that, without exception, there were significant racial differences in haemoglobin levels, at every age group, and for both sexes. This "systematic difference", the authors wrote, "is fully evident even during the period of rapid adolescent gain in haemoglobin levels in the male, and during the period of declining haemoglobin levels in the 7th and 8th decades".

Speculating on whether the observed difference in haemoglobin levels between the races was of environmental or genetic origin, the authors explained that if it were the latter, then this "would also raise the possibility of mechanisms for oxygen transport beyond those provided by the respiratory pigments". Two years later, another team of researchers, also writing in the *Journal of the National Medical Association*, reported that "some compensatory mechanism must exist to counteract this relative deficiency of haemoglobin, since a significant difference has even been demonstrated in healthy athletes".

Perhaps because the implications of lower haemoglobin levels in healthy black athletes were not fully understood, the next clue that physiological factors were primarily responsible for African-American athletic success was not uncovered for another decade. It was not until almost two decades after the authors of the Mexico City study had pointed to genetic systems related to energy metabolism as areas where explanations for differences in athletic ability might be found, that a study to determine whether there are racial differences in fibre-type proportion and how the skeletal muscles receive energy was proposed. By that time, in 1986, research over the previous decade or so had established that not only was skeletal muscle composed of two types of fibres – fast-twitch and slow-twitch – that deploy different metabolic pathways, but the proportion of those fibres influenced athletic performance.

Conducted at Laval University in Quebec, Canada, the study to determine racial differences in fibre-type proportion consisted of forty-six men: twenty-three black African students from Cameroon, Senegal, Zaire, Ivory Coast and Burundi; and an equal number of Caucasians. Since training influences enzyme activity in both fast-twitch and slow-twitch fibres, all the selected men had either never trained or had been inactive for several months. The groups were also matched by age, height, body weight and body mass index.

The study, conducted by geneticist and exercise physiologist Claude Bouchard and exercise biochemist Jean-Aimé Simoneau, revealed that the groups differed in both fibre-type proportion and muscle enzyme activity levels. Muscle biopsies clearly showed not only that the mixed group of Africans had a higher percentage of fast-twitch fibres and a lower level of slow-twitch fibres than their Caucasian counterparts, but also that the Africans had significantly higher activity, about 30 to 40 per cent, in their phosphagenic, glycolytic and lactate dehydrogenase metabolic pathways. The authors con-

cluded that "the racial differences observed between Africans and Caucasians in fibre type proportion and enzyme activities . . . may well result from inherited variation. These data suggest that sedentary male black individuals are, in terms of muscle characteristics, well endowed for sports events of short duration."

It may also be true that the study, by excluding African Americans, Afro-Caribbeans and other West African-descended groups in the diaspora, significantly underestimated the differences between Europeans and those West Africans whose ancestors had been transported across the Atlantic. Such differences may exist not only because of the eugenic effects of the slave trade, but also because there is reason to believe that not all West Africans are equally endowed with fast-twitch muscle fibre and that the ancestors of many of the most outstanding athletes of West African descent in the diaspora may have come, disproportionately, from a relatively small area of West Africa.

In addition to these natural selection processes, there is some evidence that the eugenic effect of slavery may have been aided by selective breeding. But it was natural selection and not selective breeding that was the primary eugenic agent during slavery.

Indeed, West African-descended populations in the New World are likely to have a higher percentage of fast-twitch muscle fibre and higher enzyme activity levels and, therefore, greater average athletic ability than West Africans whose ancestors did not leave the mother continent.

Pulmonary Function

A study was conducted at the State University of New York at Buffalo to "determine whether the lower FVC (forced vital capacity) observed in healthy blacks results in a ventilatory adjustment to exercise which differs from that observed in healthy Caucasians".

Eighteen white and fourteen black subjects were studied, ages eight to thirty, and were matched for sex, age, height and weight. The results confirmed that lung volumes were 10 to 15 per cent greater in white subjects than in blacks of the same sex, age and size; that there were clear differences in the breathing patterns of the two racial groups during exercise; and most surprisingly that blacks, despite their smaller lung capacity, consumed more oxygen in every phase of exercise than their white counterparts. This was possible, the researchers determined, because minute ventilation – the provision of oxygen to the total area of the lungs – was higher in blacks at all work loads and became more significant as the workload increased. Blacks, the study found, compensated for their smaller lung capacity by increasing the frequency of their breathing, which was achieved by a proportionate reduction of both the inspiratory and expiratory cycles.

Speculating on the differences in lung volume and the ventilatory response to exercise in his black and white subjects, the author pointed to a possible link with haemoglobin levels. Other researchers, he explained, had reported altered lung pressure-volume relationships in healthy black subjects with haemoglobin sickle-cell trait. While noting that there was no direct evidence of differences in lung compliance between the races, the author pointed out that "on indirect evidence in the literature, however, this possibility cannot be ruled out at this time".

Biochemical Differences

However flawed, the Laval University study provided the first evidence that there is, in fact, a compensatory mechanism to counteract the relative deficiency of haemoglobin even in healthy African-American athletes. The Laval study also made it clear that the mystery of African-American athletic dominance could be solved by a careful examination of the biological processes involved in the conferral of this compensation.

The black athlete, primarily because of a higher ratio of fast-twitch muscle fibre, will convert glucose into energy more rapidly than his white counterpart. Energy for muscle contraction, including all physical and athletic activities, is created by the breakdown of glucose by processes which result in the formation of adenosine triphosphate (ATP).

The first stage of the process, known as glycolysis, is cytosolic and produces ATP at a rate more than twice that of the second, intramitochondrial stage. The first stage is also far less efficient, producing far less energy per glucose molecule. Both black and white athletes will convert glucose to ATP by glycolysis – anaerobic metabolism (oxygen not required) – and by mitochondrial metabolism (oxygen required), but in different ratios. This difference in the relative efficiency or effectiveness of these metabolic pathways in the athletes plays a decisive role in performance and is largely responsible for the greater athletic success of African Americans and others of West African descent.

Skeletal muscle is composed of two types of fibres – slow-twitch and fast-twitch – classified by their speed of contraction, oxidative capacity, and resistance to fatigue. Slow-twitch or red fibres, with their high myoglobin content and greater oxidative capacity, generate

ATP primarily by the slow but efficient process of aerobic metabolism. In this process, oxygen, bound to haemoglobin in red blood cells, is carried to the muscles by the capillaries. Myoglobin, an iron–protein compound, is essential for the transfer of oxygen from the cell membrane to the mitochondria, where the oxygen is consumed.

In sharp contrast, fast-twitch or white fibres, with their lower myoglobin content and considerably lower oxidative capacity, are less able to utilize aerobic metabolism for the production of ATP and are therefore more dependent on glycolysis or anaerobic metabolism. This is why the ability to regenerate ATP during activities requiring short bursts of power is so physiologically meaningful.

Muscle biopsies have concluded, as stated earlier, that people of African descent have significantly higher levels of activity in their phosphagenic, glycolytic and lactate dehydrogenase metabolic pathways than their Caucasian counterparts. The production and regeneration of ATP take place in the glycolytic and phosphagenic pathways. Higher levels of activity result, therefore, not just in faster production of ATP but also in its more efficient regeneration. When ATP is depleted, it is rapidly replaced through a reaction that consumes creatine phosphate. Creatine phosphate acts like a battery, as a source for ATP energy, and recharges itself from the new ATP that is generated by cellular oxidations when the muscle is resting. Skeletal muscle converts chemical energy into mechanical work with relative efficiency; only 30 to 50 per cent is wasted as heat. As a result, even small differences in chemical energy generation are physiologically meaningful.

Faster production and increased regeneration of ATP, however, do not fully explain African-American biochemical superiority in athletic events requiring speed and power. There is also considerably greater activity in the lactate dehydrogenase pathway of people of West African descent. A primary function of this pathway is to reduce muscle fatigue by converting lactic acid back to glucose and re-feeding the muscles. This cyclic set of reactions, from muscles to liver and back to muscles, is known as the Cori cycle.

The postponement of muscle fatigue during prolonged anaerobic activity is dependent on a number of factors, the most important of which is the rate at which lactic acid is removed and reconverted to glucose. The removal of lactic acid from the muscles by the circulatory system reduces muscle fatigue, and its reconversion to glucose by the liver provides the muscles with additional supplies of energy. The rate of lactic acid removal is partially regulated by the activity of the lactate dehydrogenase metabolic pathway, which explains why increased activity in this pathway is so athletically meaningful.

The recycling of waste products, such as lactic acid, by the liver is vital to the proper functioning of the muscular and nervous systems, among others. If the glycogen reserves stored in the muscles were depleted during intense physical activity, blood glucose would become the major source of energy. This sequence could lower blood glucose levels enough to seriously compromise the nervous system. Additionally, during prolonged intense activity, if glucose is not available, muscle resorts to the use of fat for fuel, which is less efficient for combustion than carbohydrates. Consequently, an athlete engaged in fairly prolonged anaerobic activity – sprinting, for example – would be far less effective without a mechanism to increase the supply of glucose. This is what is accomplished during the Cori cycle, the cyclic set of reactions initiated by increased activity in the lactate dehydrogenase pathway.

Conclusion

It is this compelling array of somatogenetic variation, exhibited in muscle-fibre biology, biochemical metabolic pathways and pulmonary physiology, which is hypothesized to have been concentrated by natural selection over the centuries in the Afrocentric peoples displaced from West Africa to the New World, which is adduced to provide the athletic prowess so well documented in this group of descendants.

Not the least of coincidence seems to be the influence of the compensatory sickle-cell gene on oxygen transport and availability to the tissues. The reduced availability coupled with the reduced myoglobin in the preponderant fast-twitch muscle fibres, which are adapted for rapid energy (ATP) regeneration, all give a *net* outcome of muscle anatomical and biochemical advantages which proffer a superior performance in athleticism.

Acknowledgements

An earlier version of this article was originally published in the *West Indian Medical Journal* 55, no. 3 (June 2006): 205–9.

References

Ama, P.F.M., P. Lagasse, C. Bouchard and J.A. Simoneau. 1990. Anaerobic performances in black and white subjects. *Medicine and Science in Sports and Exercise* 22:508–11.

Carlson, D.G. 1984. *African fever: A study of British science, technology, and politics in West Africa, 1787–1864*. Canton, MA: Science History Publication.

Damon, A. 1966. Negro-white differences in pulmonary function (vital capacity, timed vital capacity, and expiratory flow rate). *Human Biology* 38(4): 381–93.

Davidson, B. 1970. *The African slave trade*. Boston: Little, Brown.

de Caray, A.L. 1974. *Genetic and anthropological studies of Olympic athletes*. New York: Academic Press.

Garn, S.M., and D.C. Clark. 1975. Lifelong differences in hemoglobin levels between blacks and whites. *Journal of the American Medical Association* 67:91–96.

Metheny, E. 1939. Some differences in bodily proportions between American Negro and white male college students as related to athletic performance. *Research Quarterly* 10:41–53.

Tanner, J. 1964. *Physique of the Olympic athlete*. London: George Allen and Unwin.

CHAPTER 4

White Men Can't Run

Where Is the Scientific Evidence?

ROBERT A. SCOTT AND YANNIS PITSILADIS

The twenty-ninth Olympiad in Beijing is over, and for the track events, this Olympics will be remembered most of all for the sporting achievements of sprinters from Jamaica and middle- and long-distance runners from Kenya and Ethiopia. Collectively, these three nations won 23 per cent of all the track and field medals on offer. The achievement of these sporting nations is more impressive when only the track events are considered. The success of East African athletes in distance running and the concurrent success of Jamaican athletes in sprint events will undoubtedly augment the idea of black athletic supremacy. This idea is not new and has emerged from simplistic interpretations of performances, such as those illustrated in table 4.1, combined with the belief that similar skin colour indicates similar genetics. As such, a number of studies have compared physiological characteristics between groups of black and white athletes. They have compared characteristics such as VO_2 max, lactate accumulation and running economy between groups of black and white athletes.

Black South African athletes were found to have lower lactate levels than white athletes for given exercise intensities (Weston et al. 1999). It has also been shown that the black athletes had better running economy (Weston et al. 2000) and higher fractional utilization of VO_2 max at race pace (Weston et al. 2000). It has been suggested that "if the physiological characteristics of sub-elite black African distance runners are present in elite African runners, this may help to explain the success of this racial group in distance running" (Weston et al. 2000). However, this assertion is difficult to reconcile with earlier studies, concluding that their findings were compatible with the concept that "Black male individuals are well endowed to perform in sport events of short duration" (Ama et al. 1986). This area

Table 4.1 Male World Records from 100-metre to Marathon

Distance	Athlete	Time	Ancestral Origin
100 metres	Usain Bolt (JAM)	9.58 s	West Africa
110-metre hurdles	Dayron Robles (CUB)	12.87 s	West Africa
200 metres	Usain Bolt (JAM)	19.19 s	West Africa
400 metres	Michael Johnson (USA)	43.18 s	West Africa
400 metre hurdles	Kevin Young (USA)	46.78 s	West Africa
800 metres	Wilson Kipketer (KEN)	1:41.11	East Africa
1,000 metres	Noah Ngeny (KEN)	2:11.96	East Africa
1,500 metres	Hicham El Guerrouj (MOR)	3:26.00	North Africa
One mile	Hicham El Guerrouj (MOR)	3:43.13	North Africa
3,000 metres	Daniel Komen (KEN)	7:20.67	East Africa
5,000 metres	Kenenisa Bekele (ETH)	12:37.35	East Africa
10,000 metres	Kenenisa Bekele (ETH)	26:17.53	East Africa
Marathon	Haile Gebrselassie (ETH)	2:03:59	East Africa

Note: Ancestral origin is derived from geographical and ethnic status.

of genetics is clearly confusing when studies comparing subjects of differing skin colour can conclude on the one hand that the results can explain the success of the racial group in distance events (Weston et al. 2000), and on the other hand that results were compatible with black male individuals' being suited to events of short duration (Ama et al. 1986). Such contradictions highlight the problem associated with grouping athletes based simply on skin colour. Despite these findings, assertions remain in the literature that East Africans have the "proper genes" for distance running (Larsen et al. 2003). However, it is unjustified to regard the phenomenal success of the East Africans and Jamaicans as genetically mediated; to justify this claim, one must identify the genes that are important. It is inevitable that the results of the Beijing Olympics will spark an even greater interest from scientists, the media and others to identify the biological mechanisms (including genes) responsible for this remarkably and seemingly unexplained phenomenon. Many of the scientists pursuing a biological or genetic explanation will ignore the socio-economic and cultural factors that appear to better explain this phenomenon (Scott and Pitsiladis 2007).

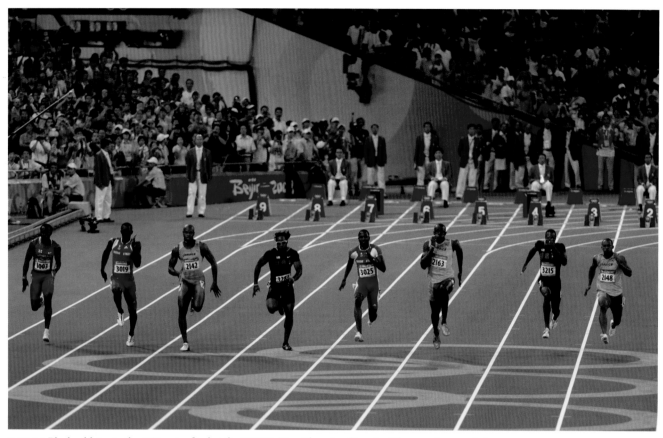

PLATE 4.1 Black athletes in the 100-metre final at the 2008 Beijing Olympics. (*Jamaica Observer* photograph.)

Non-genetic explanations for the success of East African athletes in international athletics include the suggestion that East Africans enjoy a psychological advantage, mediated through stereotype threat (Baker and Horton 2003). A consequence of strengthening the stereotypical view of the superior black or African athlete is the development of a self-fulfilling prophecy by coaches for white athletes to avoid sporting events typically considered as favouring African athletes. This self-selection has resulted in a vicious cycle where the avoidance of these athletic events by whites has further strengthened the aforementioned stereotypical view to the extent that the unsubstantiated idea of the biological superiority of the African athlete becomes dogma. This development is surprising given the lack of any scientific evidence to warrant such an assertion. Others have suggested that the distances East Africans run to school as children serve them well for subsequent athletic success. A study by Scott et al. (2003) found that elite distance runners had travelled farther to school as children, and more had done so by running. Many of the distances travelled were incredible with some children travelling upwards of twenty kilometres each day by running to and from school. A previous study by Saltin et al. (1995) has shown that East African children who had used running as a means of transport had a VO_2 max some 30 per cent higher than those who did not, therefore attributing distance travelled to school as a determinant of East African success. Other studies have shown regional disparities in the production of Ethiopian and Kenyan middle- and long-distance runners (Scott et al. 2003; Onywera et al. 2006). In a study of the demographic characteristics of elite Ethiopian athletes, 38 per cent of elite marathon athletes were from the region of Arsi, which accounts for less than 5 per cent of the Ethiopian population (Scott et al. 2003). These findings were mirrored in Kenya, where 81 per cent of international Kenyan athletes originated from the Rift Valley province, which accounts for less than a quarter of the Kenyan population (Onywera et al. 2006). Although some

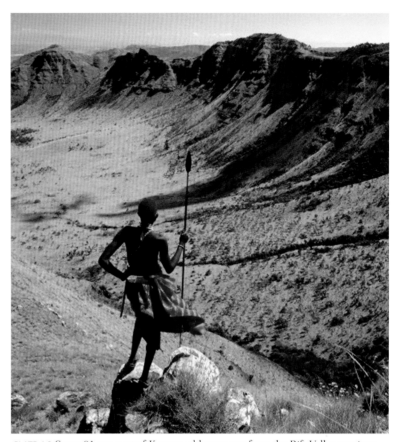

PLATE 4.2 Some 81 per cent of Kenyan athletes come from the Rift Valley province.

believe that this geographical disparity is mediated by an underlying genetic phenomenon (Manners 1997), it is worth considering that both of these regions are altitudinous (Scott et al. 2003; Onywera et al. 2006) and that athletes have long used altitude training to induce further adaptations. It has been suggested that endurance training and altitude combine synergistically in those native to moderate altitude to partially account for the success of East African athletes (Schmidt et al. 2002).

Interestingly, the vast majority of successful sprinters in Jamaica can trace their origins to the north-west region of Jamaica: the parish of Trelawny (Robinson 2007; Irving et al. forthcoming).

In the case of the Jamaican sprint phenomenon, one hypothesis proposed to explain the superior sprint performances of this population and of African Americans in general is a favourable biology concentrated by natural selection over the centuries as individuals were displaced from West Africa to the New World during the slave trade (Morrison and Cooper 2006). Morrison and Cooper (2006) posit that individuals with the sickle-cell trait possessed a significant selective advantage in the uniquely lethal West African malarial environment, and this advantage triggered a series of compensatory mechanisms producing favourable consequences for sprint/power performance. Although this hypothesis has not been rigorously tested, this idea is subject to the same limitations as genetic explanations of the East African running phenomenon, namely diverse genetic pools of founding populations and time constraints for genetic adaptations to occur.

Insight into this idea has been attempted as DNA samples from more than 120 of Jamaica's finest sprinters were collected and gene variant analysis was done for the angiotensin-converting enzyme (ACE) and actinin-3 (ACTN3). The ACE and ACTN3 genes are two of the most studied "performance genes", and both have been associated with sprint/power phenotypes and elite performance. The results of the gene variant analyses were compared with those of a large representative Jamaican control group and those of sprinters from other Caribbean islands, Nigeria and the United States (Scott et al. 2009; Irving et al. 2009).

The results showed that Jamaican athletes did not differ from controls and athletes from the other countries in their ACTN3 and ACE genotype distributions. Jamaican athletes, like control group and athletes from other countries, have a low frequency of the null variant of ACTN3 (577XX). This null variant does not produce the actinin-3 protein associated with sprinting. The results based on the ACTN3 genotype frequencies imply that very few Jamaicans, Nigerians, black Americans and Caribbean nationals are precluded from sprint success based on their ACTN3 genotype.

The phenomenal success of Jamaicans in sprinting, especially in the recent Olympics, has also been attributed to non-genetic factors. In Jamaica, there exists an excellent and unique model that focuses on identifying and nurturing athletic talent throughout junior to senior level. In his book *Jamaican Athletics: A Model for the World* (2007), Patrick Robinson concludes that "the real explanation of the outstanding achievements of the system is that all of its actors are moved by a spirit that unifies them to work to ensure that Jamaican athletics lives up to its rich history and tradition of excellence" – a theme that echoes what is found in Ethiopia and Kenya (Scott and Pitsiladis 2007). Given these unique circumstances, the superior performances of athletes from Kenya, Ethiopia and Jamaica seen in Beijing come as no surprise to those fortunate enough to study closely these amazing athletes.

The overall performances and medal tally of Team Great Britain (GB) in the Beijing Olympics may have stunned the world as much as those involved in the success. However, things are not well on the running track. The performance of Team GB in the middle- and long-distance track events is the worst in recent Olympic memory. The absence of GB athletes in the running finals in events ranging from the 1,500 to 10,000 metres in both men's and women's events was clear for all to see, as were the modest performances in both marathon races. Before the celebrations of Team GB have ended, and in preparation for London 2012 and the Commonwealth Games in Glasgow in 2014, it is hoped that those responsible for track and field will look well beyond the unfounded genetic or biological advantage of African athletes, and real efforts will be made to learn valuable lessons on how to identify and nurture athletes from these highly successful running nations.

Acknowledgements

An earlier version of this article was previously published in *Sport and Exercise Scientist* 18 (2008): 16–17.

References

Ama, P.F., J.A Simoneau, M.R. Boulay, O. Serresse, G. Theriault and C. Bouchard. 1986. Skeletal muscle characteristics in sedentary black and Caucasian males. *Journal of Applied Physiology* 61 (5): 1758–61.

Baker, J., and S. Horton. 2003. East African running dominance revisited: A role for stereotype threat? *British Journal of Sports Medicine* 37 (6): 553–55.

Irving, R., R.A. Scott, L. Irwin, E. Morrison, V. Charlton, K. Austin, S. Headley, F. Kolkhorst and Y. Pitsiladis. Forthcoming. The ACTN3 R577X polymorphism in elite Jamaican and USA sprinters. *Medicine and Science in Sports and Exercise*.

Larsen, H.B. 2003. Kenyan dominance in distance running. *Comparative Biochemistry and Physiology*, Part A: *Molecular and Integrative Physiology* 136 (1): 161–70.

Manners, J. 1997. Kenya's running tribe. *Sports Historian* 17 (2): 14–27.

Morrison, E.Y., and P.D. Cooper. 2006. Some biomedical mechanisms in athletic prowess. *West Indian Medical Journal* 55 (3): 205–9.

Onywera, V.O., R.A. Scott, M.K. Boit and Y.P. Pitsiladis. 2006. Demographic characteristics of elite Kenyan endurance runners. *Journal of Sports Sciences* 24 (4): 415–22.

Robinson, P. 2007. *Jamaican Athletics: A model for the world.* Kingston: P. Robinson.

Saltin, B., H. Larsen, N. Terrados, J. Bangsbo, T. Bak, C.K. Kim, J. Svedenhag and C.J. Rolf. 1995. Aerobic exercise capacity at sea level and at altitude in Kenyan boys: Junior and senior runners compared with Scandinavian runners. *Scandinavian Journal of Medicine and Science in Sports* 5:209–21.

Schmidt, W., K. Heinicke, J. Rojas, J.M. Gomez, M. Serrato, M. Mora, B. Wolfarth, A. Schmid and J. Keul. 2002. Blood volume and hemoglobin mass in endurance athletes from moderate altitude. *Medicine and Science in Sports and Exercise* 34 (12): 1934–40.

Scott, R.A., E. Georgiades, R.H. Wilson, W.H. Goodwin, B. Wolde and Y.P. Pitsiladis. 2003. Demographic Characteristics of elite Ethiopian endurance runners. *Medicine and Science in Sports and Exercise* 35 (10): 1727–32.

Scott, R., R. Irving, L. Irwin, M. Morrison, V. Charlton, K. Austin, D. Tladi, A. Headley, F. Kolkhorst, N. Yang, K. North and P. Pitsiladis. 2010. ACTN3 and ACE genotypes in elite Jamaican and US sprinters. *Medicine and Science in Sports and Exercise* 42 (1): 107–15.

Scott, R.A., and Y.P. Pitsiladis. 2007. Genotypes and distance running: Clues from Africa. *Sports Medicine* 37 (4): 1–4.

Weston, A.R., O. Karamizrak, A. Smith, T.D. Noakes and K.H. Myburgh. 1999. African runners exhibit greater fatigue resistance, lower lactate accumulation, and higher oxidative enzyme activity. *Journal of Applied Physiology* 86 (3): 915–23.

Weston, A.R., Z. Mbambo and K.H. Myburgh. 2000. Running economy of African and Caucasian distance runners. *Medicine and Science in Sports and Exercise* 32 (6): 1130–34.

CHAPTER 5

Physical Therapy

Keeping Athletes on the Move

SHARMELLA ROOPCHAND-MARTIN,
CARRON GORDON AND GAIL NELSON

Jamaican track and field athletes have held the spotlight in the international arena for many years. To date, track and field athletes have brought home over forty-five medals, which is a significant feat for a small country. The success of the nation's athletes over the years may be attributed to many factors, including better training facilities, better training techniques, diet and genetics. Injuries are a common occurrence in all sports, and in sprinters the majority of injuries is confined to the lower extremities, with stress fractures and hamstring strains being at the top of the list (Brukner and Kahn 2006; D'Souza 1994).

Hamstring strains have been reported to account for 50 per cent of all muscular injuries in sprinters (Arge 1985). These injuries are frustrating for both the athlete and the medical professional. The symptoms are persistent, healing is slow and the rate of re-injury is high (Petersen and Hölmich 2005). In addition, injury results in loss of time from training and competition which also translates to loss of income for many athletes and, for some, early termination of their careers.

Jamaican athletes are by no means exempt from these injuries, and data from the Jamaica Association of Sports Medicine shows that the majority of injuries occurring at the 2010 Inter-Secondary Schools Sports Association (ISSA) Boys' and Girls' Athletic Championships were of the lower limb, with hamstring injuries representing 42 per cent of injuries. The ISSA Boys' and Girls' Championships is one of the major athletic meets held annually in Jamaica and it highlights the prowess of outstanding athletes, many of whom later attain elite status.

A number of factors have been associated with the increased occurrence of hamstring injuries with the majority of the studies being conducted in soccer, Australian rules football and rugby players (Ekstrand and

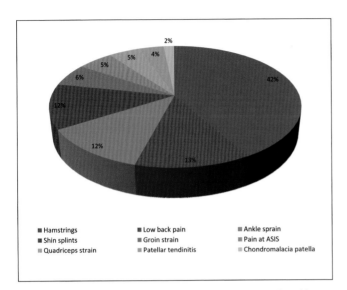

Hamstrings 42%
Low back pain 13%
Ankle sprain 12%
Shin splints 12%
Groin strain 6%
Pain at ASIS 5%
Quadriceps strain 5%
Patellar tendinitis 4%
Chondromalacia patella 2%

- Hamstrings
- Shin splints
- Quadriceps strain
- Low back pain
- Groin strain
- Patellar tendinitis
- Ankle sprain
- Pain at ASIS
- Chondromalacia patella

FIGURE 5.1: Injury statistics at the 2010 ISSA Boys' and Girls' Athletic Championships.

Gilliquist 1983; Brooks et al. 2006). These risks have been commonly divided into intrinsic (athlete-related) and extrinsic (environment-related) factors. However, a more useful classification may be to consider them as modifiable and non-modifiable risk factors (Bahr and Holme 2003). The most common non-modifiable risk factors that have been identified are older age and black or aboriginal ethnic origin (Petersen and Hölmich 2005). The most common modifiable risk factors were muscle imbalance, muscle fatigue, hamstring tightness, insufficient warm-up and previous injury (Petersen and Hölmich 2005). The literature is unclear as to which individual factor or combination of factors contributes most to the occurrence of these injuries and consequently all factors should be considered in treatment and prevention programmes. Athletes who return to sport before full recovery are at risk of recurrent and possibly more severe injury (Petersen and Hölmich 2005).

A multidisciplinary approach must be adopted in the management of athletic injuries. The team comprises the physical therapist, physician, sports medicine specialist, emergency medical technician, certified athletic trainer, sports psychologist, nutritionist, radiologist and biomechanist. During training sessions and competition, a physical therapist should be present so that injuries can be effectively managed and the athlete carefully monitored during the acute, sub-acute, remodelling, functional training and return to competition phases of injury management. In order to help an athlete reach his or her highest potential, training programmes must be individualized. Pre-participation evaluations for muscle strength, muscle endurance, flexibility and power should be conducted for each athlete and training programmes should be designed to target areas of deficits.

Due to the economic constraints experienced by many in the Jamaican context, several athletes and their coaches or teams are unable to retain the services of a physical therapist for coverage of training and competitive meets. The Jamaica Association of Sports Medicine (JASM) is the group through which most athletic teams and event organizers access physical therapy services for coverage of sporting events. They report that approximately twenty therapists regularly work with athletes (JASM Secretariat, personal communication, July 2010). This is inadequate to provide coverage for annual track meets, the various track clubs and all the high school track teams.

In many cases access to physical therapy for athletes is limited to the acute stage (the period immediately after the injury has been sustained) or when further participation in sport is jeopardized. Often, the mild injuries sustained by our future elite athletes (at the high school level) are overlooked as they continue to work through training and competition events. This can lead to compromised performance and even loss of the athlete from the sport due to more severe injuries that may occur.

Addressing Modifiable Risk Factors for Hamstring Injuries

Sprinting is a sport that requires explosive force generation. Training programmes must therefore focus on techniques that can develop muscle power while keeping in mind the specificity of training and motor learning principles. Specificity refers to the principle of directing training to performance in the athlete's given sport (Brukner and Kahn 2006). As there are many variables determining specific training effects, it is impossible to produce a general formula for training programmes. In order to help an athlete reach his or her highest potential, training programmes must be individualized. For example, where an athlete possesses a high proportion of slow twitch fibers in specific muscles, more speed-strength training and plyometrics would be needed to achieve selective hypertrophy (Delecluse 1997). Comprehensive baseline evaluations to identify modifiable risk factors must be conducted for each athlete before engaging in a training programme. This will allow for the identification of the modifiable risk factors for the athlete and, consequently, a training regime that addresses the individual's specific deficits can be developed. Likewise, it is important to complete comprehensive assessments before allowing the athlete to return to competition after treatment for injuries.

Personal communication with a therapist affiliated to one of the clubs that has consistently produced premier athletes indicates that comprehensive evaluations were done only with the elite athletes and a few of the high school athletes. This was primarily due to a lack of qualified staff to do these evaluations. With regard to post-injury management, the elite athletes would complete anywhere between 85 to 90 per cent of the rehabilitation process and return to the sport. The high school athletes, however, would, on average, complete only 15 per cent of the rehabilitation process. Cost was cited as the primary factor accounting for the differences between the two categories of athletes. Physical therapy fees for the club athletes are covered by the club. For most of the high school athletes, however, their parents or guardians are responsible for covering the cost of treatment and they are often unable to do so. The therapist interviewed also cited schoolwork and attending classes as other significant barriers to compliance with the rehabilitation process. For elite athletes, training and competing are their primary focus and when injury occurs they are more likely to comply fully with any programme that will return them to competition in the shortest possible time. On the other hand, high school athletes may have to give more focus to academic performance. A lack of understanding of the healing process could also contribute to the differences in compliance. High school athletes tend to believe that they do not need further rehabilitation once they no longer feel pain, whereas elite athletes understand that absence of pain is just the beginning of the rehabilitation process (M. Campbell, personal communication, July 2010).

Muscular Imbalance

Muscular imbalance has been identified as a modifiable risk factor for hamstring injuries, in particular the hamstring to quadriceps ratio (Petersen and Hölmich 2005). These imbalances can be assessed by using a variety of

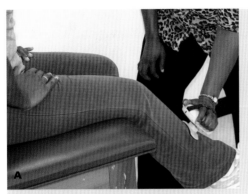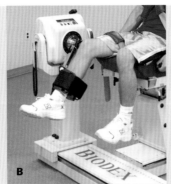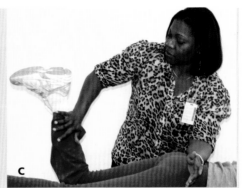

PLATE 5.1 Strength evaluation techniques: (a) manual muscle testing using a hand-held dynamometer, (b) isokinetic strength testing and (c) manual muscle testing.

muscle testing techniques. Manual muscle testing is the technique that is most commonly used by therapists in Jamaica. Hand-held dynamometers are also used by some therapists locally and these allow for detecting smaller differences in muscle imbalance. More advanced laboratory testing and training involves the use of computerized isokinetic machines, which allow for testing and training at different speeds and resistance. Currently no training or treatment facility in Jamaica has isokinetic testing equipment.

Once the pattern of imbalance is identified, several approaches to strength training, ranging from the use of free weights to use of gym equipment and aquatics, can be applied. The primary goal for sprinters is obtaining muscle hypertrophy and increased neuronal activation (Delecluse 1997). The hamstrings and quadriceps muscles should be targeted, as well as gluteus maximus and adductor magnus since these two work together with the hamstring to contribute to maximal acceleration during a sprint (Delecluse 1997). Training should concentrate on both concentric, or shortening, contractions and eccentric, or lengthening, contractions. Frequency and intensity of training should be based on the

baseline findings and the regime is developed by the therapist, coach and trainer.

In the acute stage of a hamstring injury (one to seven days) strength training is not recommended. During the sub-acute phase (three to twenty-one days), concentric training can be started when the athlete has achieved a full pain-free range of motion. Large number of sets of repetitions using submaximal loads is recommended for this. Eccentric strength training is added in the remodelling phase (seven to forty-two days).

Flexibility

Hamstring tightness is another modifiable risk factor for a hamstring strain (Petersen and Hölmich 2005). Flexibility evaluation for the hamstring can be done using a goniometer to measure extensibility of the muscle over the hip and knee joints. Global flexibility of the trunk and lower limb can be evaluated by using the modified sit-and-reach test (Minkler and Patterson 1994). There is much controversy about the role of stretching in athletic training. Some authors believe that the concept of stretching is based on intuition and

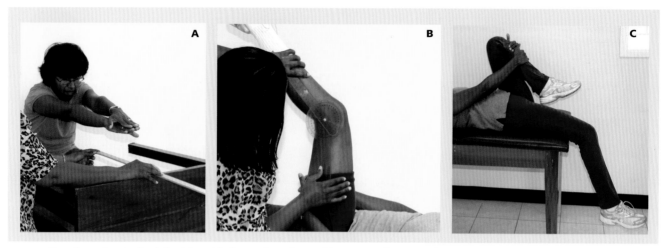

PLATE 5.2 Tests for evaluating flexibility (a) modified sit-and-reach test, (b) measuring hamstring flexibility and (c) measuring iliopsoas flexibility.

that there is no sound scientific proof to justify claims of risk reduction for injury (Thacker et al. 2004). In fact, some authors have indicated that stretching before an event may be detrimental to performance and stretching just prior to any high-energy athletic event should be avoided (Bradley et al. 2007). Generally, however, it is agreed that overall maintenance of a good level of flexibility is important for any athlete and stretching does increase flexibility and aid in recovery of muscle injuries (Malliaropoulos et al. 2004).

Muscle Fatigue

Muscle fatigue is the third modifiable risk factor that has been identified for hamstring strains (Petersen and Hölmich 2005). Two aspects of muscle function – power and muscular endurance – must be considered when assessing the risk for rapid fatigue.

Power is the product of force and velocity. There are several tests for evaluating power in runners; some are treadmill based while others are field based. One such test is the maximal anaerobic running test (MART) (Rusko et al. 1993; Nunmela et al. 1996) which requires the athlete to complete n number of 20-second runs with recovery periods of 100 seconds. Treadmill speed is increased until the athlete reaches exhaustion. Other tests for evaluating lower-limb power include the vertical jump test, which looks at how high the athlete can jump, and the standing broad-jump test, which looks at how far forward the athlete can jump.

Muscular endurance is related to the ability of the muscle to sustain a specific amount of force over a period of time. Evaluations of muscular endurance are usually based on the athlete completing as many repetitions as he or she can of a particular activity within a set period of time. Some of the tests for endurance may use external resistance while others use body weight as the resistance. Tests used to evaluate muscle endurance include the bench press, chest press, push-up and curl-up tests.

Power endurance training is more important for sprinters than strength endurance training. Exercises

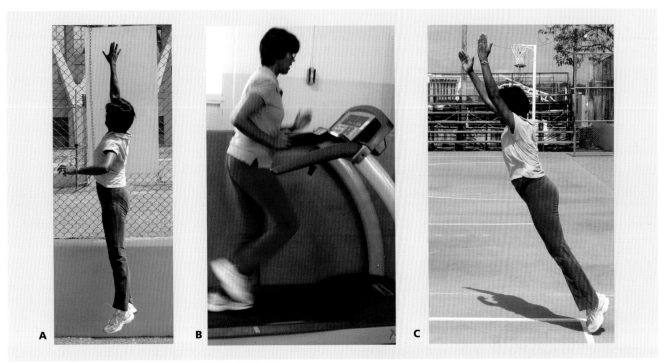

PLATE 5.3 Tests for evaluating muscle power: (a) vertical jump test, (b) anaerobic treadmill test and (c) standing broad-jump test.

such as running uphill or pulling a parachute while sprinting can be considered. Plyometric training is an interesting approach to power training that is being used in some training programmes in Jamaica. Maximal-effort plyometric training was first introduced in Russia in 1969 by Yuri Verkhoshansky to help in the development of "explosive speed strength" in sprinters. It consists of exercises involving rapid stretching of a muscle (eccentric action) followed immediately by a shortening of that same muscle (concentric action). Plyometric drills usually involve stopping, starting and changing directions in an explosive manner (Miller 2006). This type of training can be conducted effectively on land as well as in the water (Martel et al. 2005). A primary advantage of training in the water is a

reduction in the compressive forces on the load bearing joints.

Sprinting is not considered to be an endurance sport and therefore sprinters will not usually engage in aerobic training in the same manner as a marathon runner or cross-country cyclist. There is some controversy about the effects of aerobic training done concurrently with anaerobic training. Some argue that it may interfere with strength/power development while others have shown no interference effect (Kraemer et al. 1995; McCarthy, Pozinak, Agre 2002). Nevertheless, aerobic training for sprinters can be beneficial as it may confer benefits such as quicker recovery between anaerobic work intervals (repeated sprints). It may also be beneficial in maintaining optimum body weight or reducing body fat (Coburn 2000). Furthermore, aerobically trained sprinters may be better able to regulate body temperature thereby improving tolerance in hot environments (McArdle, Katch and Katch 2001). Good cardiovascular endurance is important in the maintenance of good health for everyone.

Insufficient Warm-Up

Insufficient warm-up prior to participating in a sprinting event has been shown to be a risk factor for hamstring strains (Petersen and Hölmich 2005). Adequate warm-up reduces the susceptibility to injury by increasing connective tissue extensibility, improving joint range of motion and function, and enhancing muscular performance (Pollock, Gaesser and Butcher 1998). The warm-up should consist of about five to ten minutes of low-intensity activity and may be followed by gentle stretching of major muscle groups.

Previous Injury

Having a previous hamstring injury predisposes a sprinter to a recurrent injury (Petersen and Hölmich 2005). This risk is further increased if the rehabilitation process is terminated prematurely. All injuries (minor and major) should be assessed, fully rehabilitated and thoroughly reassessed prior to allowing the athlete to return to competition. This approach is not consistently followed in Jamaica and efforts should continue to move our athletic programmes in this direction in order to optimize the athlete's performance at all levels (high school, club, national).

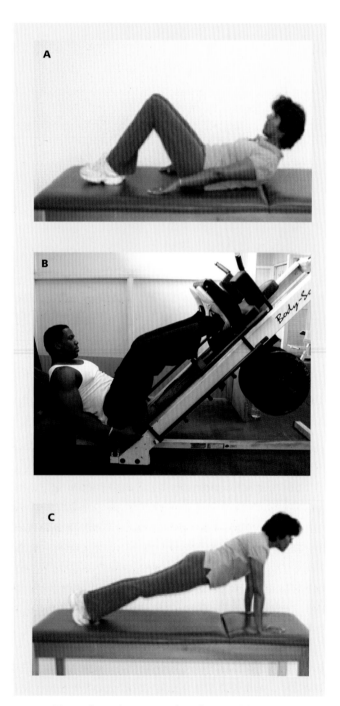

PLATE 5.4 Testing for evaluating muscle endurance: (a) curl-up test, (b) leg-press test and (c) push-up test.

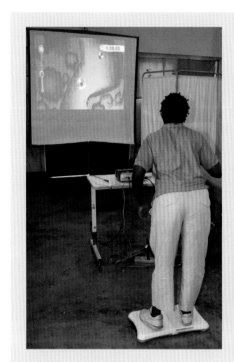
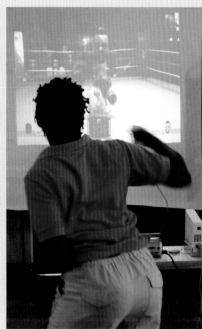
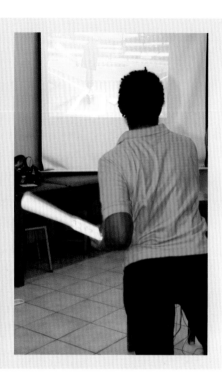

PLATE 5.5 A virtual training environment.

Future Directions and Research

Sports-related research focuses on training programmes, injury prevention and specific protocols for management of injuries. Areas of study include investigation of different training approaches and their impact on performance. Researchers spend considerable time trying to determine optimal duration, frequency and intensity for training in a variety of sports, including sprinting. Factors related to flexibility, strength, speed, power, coordination, timing and sequencing of muscle activity are just a few of the parameters that are under investigation.

A good understanding of the biomechanics of sprinting is valuable for all parties involved in sprint pro-

grammes. Today, the emergence of more sophisticated wireless technology allows for research to be conducted both on the running track and in a laboratory. Telemetric electromyography systems can be used to analyse the pattern of muscle activation of an elite sprinter during an actual sprint. Full-body wireless motion systems can be used for the precise tracking of all joint movements during an activity. The type of information that can now be acquired will help with the development of outstanding training programmes for emerging athletes.

As research progresses, virtual applications (computerized simulations) are increasingly being explored and the face of athletic training is changing. Scientific research paves the way for improving training and on-the-field injury management, and it is therefore important that sports physical therapists keep abreast of developments. The future of sprint training may one day evolve to include athletes in competition with on-the-field holograms that are constantly running at world records. Until then, Jamaica continues to dominate the athletics scene internationally and should continue to do so in the future.

References

Arge, J.C. 1985. Hamstring injuries: Proposed aetiological factors, prevention and treatment. *Sports Medicine* 2:21–33.

Bahr, R., and I. Holme. 2003. Risk factors for sports injuries: A methodological approach. *British Journal of Sports Medicine* 37:384–92.

Bradley, P.S., P.D. Olsen and M.D. Portas. 2007. The effect of static, ballistic and proprioceptive neuromuscular stretching on vertical jump performance. *Journal of Strength and Conditioning Research* 21 (1): 223–26.

Brooks, J.H., C.W. Fuller, S.P. Kemp et al. 2006. Incidence, risk and prevention of hamstring muscle injuries in professional rugby union. *American Journal of Sports Medicine* 34:1297–306.

Brukner, P., and K. Khan. 2006. *Clinical sports medicine.* 3rd ed. Sydney: McGraw Hill.

Coburn, J. 2000. Concurrent strength and endurance training for strength/power athletes. National Strength and Conditioning Association. http://www.nsca_lift.org (12 July 2010).

Delecluse, C. 1997. Influence of strength training on sprint running performance. *Sports Medicine* 24 (3): 147–56.

D'Souza, D. 1994. Track and field athletics injuries: A one-year survey. *British Journal of Sports Medicine* 28:197–202. http:// bjsm.bmj.com (4 May 2009).

Ekstrand, J., and J. Gilliquist. 1983. Soccer injuries and their mechanism: A prospective study. *Medicine and Science in Sports and Exercise* 15:267–70.

Kraemer, W.J., J.F. Patton, S.E. Gordon, E.A. Harman et al. 1995. Compatibility of high intensity strength and endurance training on hormonal and skeletal muscle adaptation. *Journal of Applied Physiology* 78 (3):976–89.

Malliaropoulous, N., S. Papalexandris, A. Papalada and E. Papacostas. 2004. The role of stretching in rehabilitation of hamstring injuries: 80 athletes follow-up. *Medicine and Science in Sports and Exercise.* http://wwwacsm.msse.org (3 May 2009).

Martel, G.F., M. Harmer, J.M. Logan and C.B. Parker. 2005. Aquatic plyometric training increases vertical jump in female volleyball players. *Medicine and Science in Sports and Exercise* 10:1814–19.

McArdle, W.D., F.I. Katch and V.L. Katch. 2001. Exercise physiology: Energy, nutrition and human performance. 5th ed. Philadelphia: Lippincott, Williams and Wilkins.

McCarthy, J., M.A. Pozniak and J.C. Agre. 2002. Neuromuscular adaptations to concurrent strength and endurance training. *Medicine and Science in Sports and Exercise* 34 (3): 511–19.

Miller, M.G., J.J. Herniman, M.D. Ricard, C.C. Cheatham and T.J. Michael. 2006. The effects of a 6-week plyometric training program of agility. *Journal of Sports Science and Medicine* 5:459–65. http://jssm.org (3 May 2009).

Minkler, S., and P. Patterson. 1994. The validity of the modified sit and reach test in college-age students. *Research Quarterly in Exercise and Sports* 65:189–92.

Nunmela, A., M. Alberts, R.P. Rijntjes, P. Luhtanen and H. Rusko. 1996. Reliability and validity of the maximal anaerobic running test. *International Journal of Sports Medicine* 17. Suppl. no. 2:97–102.

Petersen, J., and P. Hölmich. 2005. Evidence based prevention of hamstring injuries in sport. *British Journal of Sports Medicine.* 39:319–23.

Pollock, M.L., G.A. Gaesser and J.D. Butcher. 1998. ACSM position stand: The recommended quantity and quality of exercise for developing and maintaining cardiorespiratory and muscular fitness and flexibility in healthy adults. *Medicine and Science in Sports and Exercise* 30:975–91.

Rusko, H., A. Nunmela and A. Mero. 1993. A new method for the evaluation of anaerobic running power in athletes. *European Journal of Applied Physiology* 66:97–101.

Thacker, S.B., J. Gilchrist, D.F. Stroup and C.D. Kimsey. 2004. The impact of stretching on sports injury risk: A systematic review of the literature. *Medicine and Science in Sports and Exercise.* http://www.acsm.msse.org (3 May 2009).

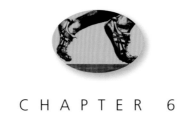

CHAPTER 6

Jamaican Yams, Athletic Ability and Exploitability

The word *yam* is one of a few words of West African origin to have entered the English language. It is believed to have been derived from the Mande *niam* or the Temne *enyame*. This was then adopted into the Portuguese language as *ynhame*, Spanish as *name*, French as *igname* and finally into English as *yam*. The term "yam" has been misapplied to almost any edible starchy root, tuber or rhizome grown in the tropics. In the United States, "yam" usually refers to the sweet potato. Yams are also often confused with a number of edible tubers such as cocoyams, taros, dasheens, eddoes, tanias or yautias. Due to the misapplication of the term "yam", it has been suggested that the term be reserved for the economically useful plants or tubers of the genus Dioscorea. In recognition of this, many people refer to tubers of the genus Dioscorea as the "true yam".

Yam is a monocotyledonous, tuber-bearing plant. Tubers vary in shape, numbers and forms, depending

on the yam species. The fresh weight of the yam tubers usually ranges from 2 to 50 kilograms, depending on the species or agricultural practice. The yam plant consists of three morphological regions: shoot, roots and tuber or bulbils. Vines of many species are armed with

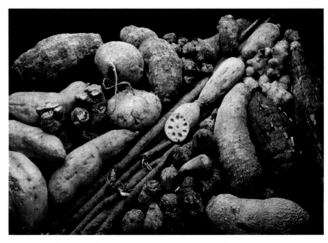

PLATE 6.1 "Yam" has been misapplied to almost all edible starchy roots, tubers or rhizomes.

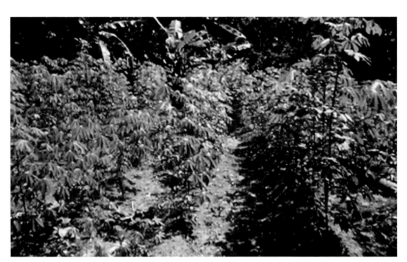

PLATE 6.2 Young yam vines.

Jamaican Yams

In Jamaica, there are over twenty-four local cultivars of yams belonging to the six economically cultivated species. The common names of some of these cultivars are roundleaf yellow yam, Lucea yam, Negro yam, St Vincent yam, Chinese yam, white yam and sweet yam. There are also the inedible yams which are referred to as "wild yams". They are usually found in the wild and grow mainly in the limestone regions of the island. A typical example is the bitter yam.

White yam originated in West Africa and is considered to be one of the four most important yam varieties in that region, as it is thought to be the best for making dough for "fufu". The white yams store better than the yellow yams and are more tolerant to the long dry season typical of West Africa. They are also known by a host of local names and are quite similar to water yams but more solid.

Yellow yams are indigenous to the forest zone of West Africa, which has a short dry season. It requires a full

spines which provide support in twining and act as a deterrent to animal predators. The length of the vine varies with species, from short in dwarf species to several metres in others. Most yam species have cylindrical or circular vines, while some vines are rectangular or polygonal in cross section. The leaves which are borne on the vines are petiolate and vary in shape depending on the species. Most yam leaves are heart-shaped and simple, but a few have lobed leaves and are generally pointed at the tips.

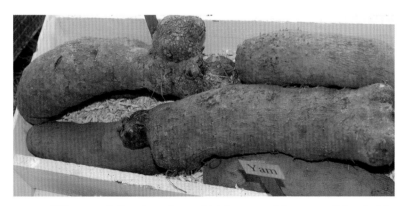
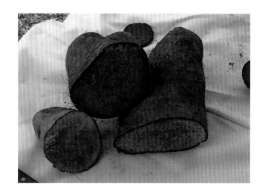

PLATE 6.3 Yellow yam (*left*) and purple yam (*right*) are two of the most well-loved of the twenty-four local cultivars of yams in Jamaica.

year for maturity and is considered one of the most important yam types in the world.

The greater yam, or Asiatic yam, is believed to have originated and to have been first cultivated in Southeast Asia. It requires at least 60 inches of rain per year and is the highest yielding of the yam crops. The white, brown or brownish red root tubers are very large, sometimes over 2 metres in length, and penetrate deep into the soil. Tubers can weigh up to 130 pounds and take ten months to a year to mature, and usually keep well for five to six months after harvest.

Cush-cush yam is the only yam indigenous to northern South America but is now widely grown in the Caribbean. It is called "yampie" and by many other local names, depending on the country. This yam bears clusters of up to a dozen tubers of good quality and is the only species with both lobed leaves and a winged stem. It is small and elongated with charcoal to purplish skin that is lightly striated but fairly smooth.

Jamaican Yam Cultivation

Traditional yam cultivation involves the use of the edible yam tubers as planting materials, which results in a considerable amount of the harvested tuber's being reserved for planting the next growing season. The basic principle behind the use of the tuber as planting material is that it sprouts readily. If the tuber is in a moist medium, the bud will immediately proceed to elongate, and a ring of stout roots will form at the junction of the bud with the tuber. When the bud has elongated to become a vine, its junction with the roots and the old tuber remains attached to the new tuber. Thus the yam head is the source of roots, shoots and tubers during sprouting. The multiplicity of the tuber planting mate-

rial is very low as one tuber head, when planted, usually results in one plant.

There have been a number of attempts to improve cultivation practices through the introduction of the minisett technique and, to a lesser extent, tissue culture. Minisett involves the cutting of the whole tuber into six to eight pieces, resulting in only six to eight plants. The use of tuber pieces in minisett has shown that small setts usually result in low yields per sett at harvest time. This reduces the amount available for consumption and export.

Yam propagation by tissue culture offers the ultimate in clonal multiplication. From a single tuber block of nodal section, it is theoretically possible to produce millions of little yam plants within a single year. It is, therefore, a method that offers promise when rapid multiplication of a single desirable plant is required. The plantlets produced by tissue culture can then be grown to maturity and their tubers planted again.

Yam as Food

Edible yam tubers act as a primary source of energy to millions of people in Africa, Southeast Asia (including Japan and parts of China), the Pacific and the Caribbean. In many parts of Nigeria, yams are usually peeled, boiled and pounded in a wooden mortar to yield glutinous dough commonly called "fufu" or pounded yam. However, only some varieties are suitable for pounding or mashing after cooking, while the others are eaten boiled, roasted, baked or fried. Yam is also used to make flour by grinding dried pieces of the tuber and is used in preparation of composite flour with cereal for use in baking. The yam flour or mashed yam is also used as a thickener in soups, particularly afia efere, or "white soup". Mashed boiled yams are used to make yam balls, which are usually fried before consumption. In Jamaica, yams are traditionally consumed boiled or roasted (cooking on an open flame).

The food value of yams is based on the carbohydrate, protein, amino acid, vitamin and mineral content. The amount of lipids is negligible in terms of food value. The proximate composition of edible yam tuber is water (65–75 per cent), carbohydrates (mainly starch; 15–25 per cent), protein (1–2.5 per cent), fibre (0.5–1.5 per cent), minerals (0.7–2.0 per cent) and fat (0.05–0.20 per cent). Yams have shown wide variation in mineral content, with calcium content 12.0–69.00 mg/100 g, phosphorus 17–61 mg/100 g, iron 0.7–5.2 mg/100 g, sodium 8–12 mg/100 g and potassium 294–397 mg/100 g tuber dry weight. Reports have shown variations in vitamin contents with ß-carotene equivalence of 0–10 mg/100 g, thiamine 0.01–0.11 mg/100 g, riboflavin 0.01–0.04 mg/100 g, niacin 0.3–0.8 mg/100 g, nicotinic acid 0.07–1.07 mg/100 g, dehydroascorbic acid 7.3–7.6 mg/100 g and ascorbic acid 4.0–18.0 mg/100 g, with total vitamin C of 17–27.6 mg/100 g tuber on a dry weight basis. It has been shown that the quantity of yam consumed daily per person (0.5–1 kg) can supply the requirements of vitamin C. Most yams tend to be deficient in fat-soluble vitamins, which is primarily due to the low lipid content of the tubers. It has been reported that the tubers of bitter yam tend to be richer in most vitamins than the commonly edible species. Yams also have high amounts of essential amino acids, which include arginine (300 mg/gN), histidine (106–125 mg/gN), isoleucine (181–281 mg/gN), leucine (344–588 mg/gN), lysine (263–300 mg/gN), phenylalanine (238–344 mg/gN), tyrosine (181–300 mg/gN), cystine (0–113 mg/gN), methionine (63–112 mg/gN), threonine (0–294 mg/gN), tryptophan (188–294

mg/gN) and valine (250–369 mg/gN). Yams are generally thought of as a good source of native starches which have varying functional characteristics and could find some application in the food ingredients industry.

Non-food Industrial Applications

Over 250,000 tonnes of yams are produced annually in Jamaica; however, only about 5 per cent is exported, with losses of up to 40 per cent of the total production reported. These losses are primarily because the yam tubers cannot be stored for longer periods. The loss can be prevented if their starches are extracted and industrially exploited immediately after harvest. Presently, yams are not listed among the most common sources of industrial starch, which is primarily met by corn, potato, wheat, tapioca and rice.

Within the European Union, the industrial starch market amounts to 2.4×10^6 tonnes per annum. The United Kingdom's industrial use accounts for 2.2×10^5 tonnes, which is over 25 per cent of the total starch used in the United Kingdom. Developed countries such as Canada, the United States, Europe and Japan utilize over 77 per cent of the starch globally. Of the world starch production, the food sector alone consumes over 55 per cent, whereas the other 45 per cent is utilized in the board industries in textile, adhesive, glue and pharmaceutical products. There are strong implications that Jamaican yam starches can be exploited for their industrial applications, particularly in the pharmaceutical industry in the formulation of capsules and tablets.

Yam as Medicine

The wild yam has been used in traditional medicine in Africa for hundreds of years as a treatment for rheuma-

Table 6.1 Industrial Uses of Starch

Industry	Use of Starch/Modified Starch
Adhesive	Adhesive production
Agrochemical	Mulches, pesticide delivery, seed coatings
Cosmetics	Face and talcum powders
Detergent	Surfactants, builders, co-builders, bleaching agents, bleaching activators
Food	Viscosity modifier and glazing agent
Medical	Plasma extenders/replacers, transplant organ preservation, absorbent sanitary products
Oil drilling	Viscosity modifier
Paper and board	Binding, sizing and coating
Pharmaceuticals	Diluent, binder, filler, disintegrants, drug delivery
Plastics	Biodegradable filler
Purification	Flocculants
Textile	Sizing, finishing and printing, fire resistance

tism and arthritis-like ailments. Fresh tubers of yams have been found to consist of two important classes of metabolites, namely alkaloids and steroids. These metabolites are thought to be responsible for the herb-like taste of the tubers. Wild yams are good sources of steroidal precursors, and most species contain large amounts of plant steroids such as diosgenin (a saponin), which acts as a precursor in the synthesis of progesterone used in the manufacture of oral contraceptives. Bitter yam tubers have been used in the treatment of tropical diseases, such as leprosy and tumours.

Yam tubers have also been used as phytotherapeutic agents for the treatment of diabetes and as anaesthetics. Infertility has been reported to have been minimized by the use of yam tubers. Yam tubers are also employed in certain ayurvedic (the ancient Hindu science of health and medicine) preparations recommended for piles and dysentery. Wild yam tubers have been shown to contain high levels of dehydroepiandosterone, commonly known as DHEA, which is identical to a hormone produced in the adrenal glands of mammals. DHEA is the most abundant steroid circulating in the plasma of normal human adults. Reports by the British Herbal Medicine Association characterize the wild yam tuber as a spasmolytic, mild diaphoretic, anti-inflammatory, anti-rheumatic and cholagogue, for use in the treatment of intestinal cholic, rheumatoid arthritis, muscular rheumatism, diverticulitis, dysmenorrhoea, intermittent claudication, cholecystitis, cramps, and ovarian and uterine pain. Wild yam has also shown cardioprotective effects, including increasing beneficial high density lipids (HDL), reducing triglycerides and reducing blood fats.

Yam and Athletic Disposition Propaganda: The True Scenario

Jamaica's above-par performance at the Beijing Olympics has attracted international interest with many persons now vying to unravel the secret of the success of the Jamaican athletes. It is thought that many persons in the mainstream media have begun to attribute their success overwhelmingly to yam consumption, because of the athletes' yam-rich diet. As a result, yam is now dubbed "the speed agent". The basis of yam being called so is one which is not entirely clear, but several schools of thought prevail. One perspective is based on the fact that a large percentage of Jamaica's top athletes are from the Cockpit region of the country, where yam is widely grown and consumed. Their athletic prowess could, therefore, be attributed to their yam-rich diet. Without scientific proof, this remains just a guess at best. Within this school of thought, however, there lies a more plausible explanation, which is still only a hypothesis, from our perspective. The phytosterols in yams have the potential to stimulate cell growth and as such may be responsible for enhanced stimulation of proteins essential to muscle function, including proteases, lactate dehydrogenase and actinin-3 protein, which are a part of fast-twitch muscle fibres. Activation of these fast-twitch fibres could in turn cause improvements in muscle speed and overall power. The possibility and rate of this happening has yet to be unravelled. Studies have shown that more than 6 per cent of all prescriptions in human medicine are steroidal hormones. Diosgenin, a saponin derivative of yams, is of great interest as it is easily converted into the starting material for synthesis of these steroidal hormones. Could it be that the presence of phytosterols in yams may indirectly result in enhanced muscle mass and speed?

The use of the glycemic index (GI) concept also has strong implications in the sporting arena, where athletes can utilize the GI concept to optimize their performance. GI is a measure of how rapidly a carbohydrate is absorbed into the bloodstream. It is based on a numerical scale between 1 and 100. Foods are classified as having a low, moderate or high glycemic response based on where they fall on the scale, and GI can be used to gauge how a particular food, or combinations of foods, will affect blood sugar and thus energy levels. Glucose directly fuels the muscles, brain and nervous systems of athletes at all stages of exercise (before, during and after). The quicker a carbohydrate becomes glucose, the faster the blood sugar will rise. Higher GI foods will raise blood sugar more quickly and to a greater extent than lower GI foods. Higher blood sugar means that more insulin will be secreted, pulling the glucose into working muscles and organs, and providing them with energy. Low to moderate GI foods are recommended when the need for rapid energy infusion is low, such as during long distance events or at mealtimes when all the other nutritional needs of an athlete are being met.

Consequently, the University of the West Indies Yam Research Group is at the forefront of this research in the Caribbean, having created a database of the GI of commonly eaten carbohydrate-rich foods indigenous to the Caribbean. This GI database consists of different varieties of yams which were found to have intermediate to high GI values; for example, yellow yam is found to have an intermediate GI, while white yam has a high GI.

The Jamaican Situation and Possibilities

In reality, the Jamaican situation relies heavily on genetics. Jamaicans are mostly derived from a West African population which expresses specific genes that result in increased power and speed of response in muscles. This feature, along with development of positive athletic attributes through proper training and maintenance programmes, may have resulted in athletes who have always been world-leading competitors. Muscles used in running are made up of a mixture of both slow-twitch and fast-twitch fibres. Research has shown that Jamaican sprinters have an above-average presence of the gene that produces actinin-3, which is an important protein for fast-twitch fibres. This is obviously desirable for sprinters. The next plausible step is to figure out if this gene can be somehow forcibly expressed, hence increasing the amounts of actinin-3, which will in turn cause the fast-twitch muscle fibres to be more efficient.

Research done at the University of the West Indies, Mona, laboratories (by Professor Asemota and co-workers) has revealed that some yams are storehouses of phytosterols and steroidal saponin precursors that support the endocrine and immune systems. Some Jamaican yam tubers contain up to 13 per cent diosgenin, which, useful in the regulation of metabolism, has been proven to have some control on infertility and is known to provide the steroid building-blocks for developing muscle mass and strength. A combination of genetic factors and phytosterols from yams may be playing a crucial role in the success of local Jamaican athletes. The actual scientifically validated link between yams and athletic prowess (now in the limelight) needs to be more fully explored for certainty. The necessary foundation data relating to yams and the capacity to do this study exist at the University of the West Indies, Mona, and should be exploited for national and global development.

Acknowledgements

The author wishes to acknowledge the following members of the Yam Research Group at the University of the West Indies, Mona: Andrew Wheatley, Lowell Dilworth, Percival Bahadosingh, Cliff Riley and Alexia Harvey.

References

Adams, C.D. 1972. *Flowering plants of Jamaica*. Glasgow: Robert MacLehose and Co., and The University Press, Glasgow.

Asemota, H.N. 1994. Biotechnological advances towards improved yam production and storage. In *Advances in tissue culture for improved planting material,* ed. K. Wood, 106–30. Kingston: Scientific Research Council.

Asemota, H.N., O.A. Iyare, A.O. Wheatley and M.H. Ahmad. 1997. Acclimatization of in vitro grown yam (Dioscorea spp.) plantlets and some enzyme changes. *Tropical Agriculture* 74:243–47.

Asemota, H.N., and A.U. Osagie. 1987. Carbohydrate metabolism in stored yam tubers: Contribution of starch breakdown, gycolysis and pentose phosphate pathway. *Advances in Yam Research* 11:67–72.

Asemota, H.N., M.A. Wellington, A. Odutuga and M. Amad. 1992. Effect of short term storage on phenolic content, O-diphenolase and peroxidase activities of cut yam tubers (Dioscorea spp.). *Journal of the Science of Food and Agriculture* 60:309–12.

Ayensu, E.S. 1972. Dioscoreales. In *Anatomy of the monocotyledons*, vol. 6, ed. C.R. Metcalfe. Oxford: Clarendon Press.

British Herbal Medicine Association (BHMA). Scientific Committee. 1983. *British herbal pharmacopoeia. Bournemouth*: BHMA.

Bahado-Singh, P.S., A.O. Wheatley, A.U. Osagie, M. Boyne, E. Choo-Kan, E.Y.StA. Morrison, M.H. Ahmad and H.N. Asemota. 2006. Effect of low glycemic index foods in the management of type 2 diabetes in the Caribbean. *West Indian Medical Journal* 55 (suppl.): 41–42.

Coursey, D.G. 1967a. Post-harvest problems of the yams (Dioscorea). In *Proceedings of the First International Sympoisium on Tropical Root Crops*. St Augustine, Trinidad.

———. 1967b. *Yams*. London: Longmans.

———. 1967c. Yam storage, I: A review of yam storage practices and of information on storage losses. *Journal of Stored Products Research* 2 (3): 229–44.

Jamaica Exporters Association (JEA). 2000. *Annual report 2000*. Kingston: JEA.

Food and Agriculture Organisation (FAO). 2002. *The state of food insecurity in the world 2002*. Rome: FAO Corporate Document Repository.

Kenyon, L. 2001. An overview of viruses infecting yams in sub-Saharan Africa. *First Symposium of Plant Virology for Sub-Saharan Africa* (PVSSA). Ibadan, Nigeria: IITA.

Muzac-Tucker, I., H.N. Asemota and M.H. Ahmad. 1993. Biochemical composition and storage of Jamaican yams (Dioscorea spp.). *Journal of the Science of Food and Agriculture* 62:219–24.

Nakanishi, K. 1974. *Natural products chemistry*, vol. 1. New York: Academic Press.

Osagie, A.U. 1992. The yam tuber in storage: An up-to-date review of the biochemical composition and storage of the yam tuber. Post Harvest Research Unit, Department of Biochemistry, University of Benin.

Onwueme, I.C. 1975. Temperature effects on yam sprouting. *Proceedings of the Agricultural Society of Nigeria* 12:18.

———. 1978. *The tropical tuber crisis: Yams, cassava, sweet potato and cocoyams*. Chichester: John Wiley and Sons.

Purseglove, J.W. 1972. *Tropical crops: Monocotyledons*. London: Longman.

Riley, C.K., A.O. Wheatley, A.S. Adebayo, M.H. Ahmad, E.Y. StA. Morrison and HN. Asemota. 2006. Effect of micrometric properties on the in vitro digestibility of starches extracted from yams (Dioscorea spp.) grown in Jamaica. *West Indian Medical Journal* 55:42.

Riley, C.K., A.S. Adebayo, A.O. Wheatley and H.N. Asemota. 2006. Exploitation of Jamaican yam starches in the pharmaceutical industry for sustainable and economic development. *Proceedings of the Twentieth Scientific Research Council Annual National Conference on Science and Technology*. Kingston, Jamaica.

Treche, S. 1989. *Potentialités nutritionnelles des ignames (Dioscorea spp.) cultivées au Cameroun*. [Nutritional potential of yams (Dioscorea spp.) cultivated in Cameroon]. Paris: Orstom éditions.

SECTION 2

Brand Jamaica:
The Lives of Some Sprinters

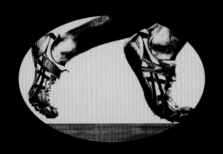

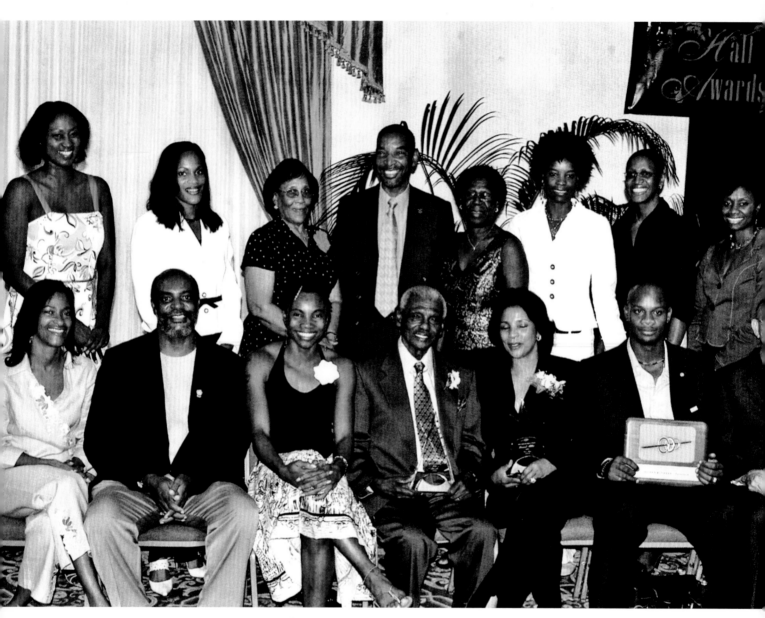

PLATE 7.1 From left, standing, are Grace Jackson, Brigitte Foster-Hylton, Carmen Laing, Clifton Forbes, Vilma Charlton, Juliet Campbell, Deon Hemmings-McCatty, Juliet Cuthbert; seated are Cathy Rattray-Williams, Anthony Davis, Aleen Bailey, Leslie Laing, Avril Miller (wife of Lennox Miller), Asafa Powell and Keith Gardner.

CHAPTER 7

A Historic Picture . . .
Tells a Fine Story

JIMMY CARNEGIE

The photograph shown on the facing page was taken on 4 November 2005 at the Jamaica session of the Central American and Caribbean Athletic Federation's Hall of Fame Induction. Keith Gardner, Les Laing and the late Dr Lennox Miller were inducted as Jamaica's latest representatives in the Hall. Vilma Charlton, president of the Olympians Association of Jamaica, thought it would be a good idea to take a picture of the Jamaican track-and-field Olympians present along with Mrs Avril Miller, Lennox's widow, who, although not an athlete herself, was indispensable in making possible a certain piece of history.

As it turned out, the athletes in the picture (with the nine ladies and Mrs Miller also providing quite a spectacular collective example of Jamaican womanhood) represented all seven decades of Jamaica's Olympic competition, from 1948 to 2004, with team members from fourteen of the fifteen Games in which Jamaica has participated during that time, the only unrepresented Games being Montreal in 1976, the eighth or "middle" one in which Jamaica participated.

As the saying goes, a picture is worth a thousand words, and a book could probably be written on this one, but this article will have to do for the moment. From the left, we start with our tallest female track Olympian, Grace Jackson, a three-timer at the Games of 1984, 1988 and 1992. In 1984 she became one of the few athletes, from any country, to run in four separate finals at one Games – the 100 metres, 200 metres and both relays. In 1988 she became the first Olympic silver medallist from the female cohort of English-speaking Caribbean sportswomen, in the 200 metres; she again pioneered the females from the region when she took sixth place in the 200 metres in the 1992 Olympics, her third straight 200-metre final, along with Juliet Cuthbert, the silver medallist, and Merlene Ottey, the bronze medallist. Jamaica had all three athletes as finalists in the same Olympic event, a feat bettered only by George Rhoden's gold, Herb McKenley's silver and Arthur Wint's fifth place in the 400-metre event in 1952.

Next to Grace is Brigitte Foster-Hylton, who is still a work in progress as a 2000/2004 Olympian in the 100-metre hurdles. At Sydney in 2000 she was a finalist and fell when she would have been a medallist, possibly even the gold medallist. The talent pool in her event may also be even deeper than Grace's own.

Coming across to the right beside Brigitte is Carmen Laing, formerly Phipps, wife of Leslie Laing and a finalist in the long jump at the 1948 Olympics. They were and are the first of three such couples who were or would be married while they were Jamaican track-and-field Olympians(the others being Raymond Stewart and Beverly McDonald, and Davian Clarke and Lacena Golding). Mrs Laing is the senior lady in the picture. Seated in front of her is Aleen Bailey of the 2004 team, the junior lady in the picture, with a gap in ages of about half a century. In addition to this, both ladies have brothers prominent in different areas of Jamaican life. In Mrs Laing's case, her brother, Hon. Frank Phipps, is one of Jamaica's most distinguished legal luminaries; in Miss Bailey's case, her brother is the DJ Capleton, as known for offering "fire fe dem" as his sister has become known for burning up the track.

Beside Mrs Laing and in the middle of the seven striking ladies in the back row is the late Clifton Forbes, captain of the 1968 athletics team in Mexico City, who after breaking George Rhoden's national (and, when set, world) record in the 400 metres with 45.7 seconds, went on to run the third leg on the sprint relay team anchored by Dr Miller. Michael Stewart and Errol Fray ran the first two legs; they first equalled and then set new world and Olympic records on the same day – only the second time that this has ever happened and the

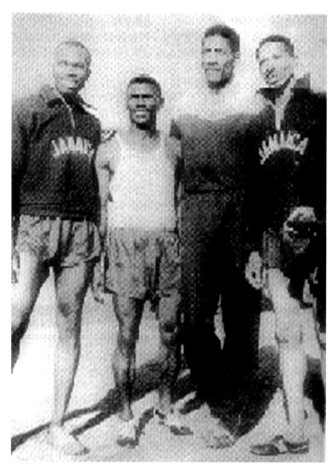

PLATE 7.2 From left to right, George Rhoden, Les Laing, Arthur Wint and Herb McKenley. Their record breaking run in the 4 × 400-metre relay at the 1952 Helsinki Olympic Games.

first time it had happened at the Games. Interestingly, sitting in front of Forbes is Les Laing, one of the honorees and a member of the immortal 1952 Helsinki 4 × 400-metre quartet which had also run in 1948 and which set world and Olympic records in winning the gold medals, the three giants Arthur Wint, Herb McKenley and George Rhoden being the other members. One more important thing resulted after the 1968 effort, in that, as a result of the world records, Jamaica became, and remains, the only country apart from the United States to hold the world records in both male Olympic relay events.

Standing beside Clifton Forbes is Vilma Charlton, a teammate from 1968 and first president of the Olympians Association of Jamaica. A good sprinter who was also a member of the 1964, 1968 and 1972 teams, she thus became, along with her good friend Una Morris (another doctor), the first three-time Jamaican female Olympian.

To Vilma's left, is Juliet Campbell, one of the few top-class all-round female sprinters Jamaica has produced. Over the 100 metres, 200 metres and 400 metres, her Olympic representation was on the fifth placed 4 × 100-metre relay team at Barcelona and at the Centennial Games, the 1996 Atlanta Olympics. She was a member of the 4 × 400-metre relay squad which finished fourth after finishing fifth in the previous three Games' finals.

To Juliet's left is probably the most historic figure in this historic picture, Deon Hemmings-McCatty. She, of course, was the first female Olympic champion, not just from Jamaica but also from the entire English-speaking Caribbean, in winning the 400-metre hurdles at the 1996 Atlanta Olympics. She also did something that the regional Olympic champions in the sport had done or were to do (before her, countrymen Arthur Wint, George Rhoden, Donald Quarrie, Hasely Crawford of Trinidad and Tobago, and two after her, Veronica Campbell-Brown of Jamaica and Tonique Williams-Darling of the Bahamas): she broke the Olympic record in the event in both the semi-final and the final. In 2000 at Sydney four years later, Hemmings-McCatty, who had finished seventh in the event at her first Games in 1992, won the silver medal to make herself the best overall record holder in the event.

Sitting in front of her is Asafa Powell, the North and Central America and the Caribbean Area Association's male athlete of the year for 2005, with his new historic world record in the 100 metres of 9.77 seconds, then only the second man to run legally under 9.80 seconds. Powell was also the fourth man from outside the United States and the first from outside the North Atlantic "metropole" to set a new record in this event, one of the two Blue Riband events in the sport, along with the men's 1,500 metres.

The last lady in the back row of the picture, standing, fittingly, beside Hemmings-McCatty, is Juliet Cuthbert, a team member in the 1980 Games and a competitor in all the other Games up to 1996. She was one of Jamaica's first two five-time female Olympians and was also the first female sportswoman from the English-speaking Caribbean region to win two silver medals (in the 100 metres and 200 metres), and to do so at the same Games (Barcelona in 1992).

Sitting in front of her is one of the honorees, Keith Gardner, vice-president of the Olympians Association of Jamaica, who, at the 1960 Rome Olympics, became the first regional Olympian to make it to the 110-metre hurdles final (and the only one for forty-four years). He was also the first, and still only, male high hurdler to win a relay medal, a bronze, in the 4 × 400-metre relay.

Moving to the front row, at left is another multiple female Olympian who, like Juliet Cuthbert, was a fifteen- or sixteen-year-old non-competitor in 1980 and then was a regular member of the female 4 × 400-metre relay teams which consistently finished fifth on all three occasions in 1984, 1988 and 1992 – Cathy Rattray Williams.

Next in line is Anthony Davis, in a sense a forerunner of Asafa Powell, as a home-grown sprinter who was part of the Olympic team – in his case as a relay reserve who, like Rattray-Williams and Cuthbert, did not compete at Moscow in 1980.

Beside Davis and moving to the right is Aleen Bailey, who after finishing fifth in the Athens 2004 final in the 100 metres (one of all three Jamaicans to do so), and fourth in the 200 metres, ran the third leg on the team which won the gold in the 4 × 100-metre relay, following Tayna Lawrence and Sherone Simpson and preceding Veronica Campbell-Brown. At age twenty-five, the youngest woman in the picture, she helped make Jamaica one of only half a dozen or so countries to win both a men's and women's relay event at the Olympic Games.

Fittingly, sitting in the centre of the picture beside Aleen Bailey is a member of that other historic relay team, the oldest man in the picture, eighty-one-year-old Leslie Laing, who was also the first non-US athlete to make it to two Olympic 200-metre finals. Along with Arthur Wint, Herb McKenley and George Rhoden, a full-strength US team was beaten in this event in head-to-head competition as Jamaica became, and still remains to date, the only non-US team in the history of the Games to set a world record in this event. He also helped, in 1948, to make Jamaica, beside the United States, the only country to have two finalists in both the 200 metres and 400 metres, and in 1952, again apart from the United States, the only country to have finalists in the 100 metres, 200 metres, 400 metres and 800 metres, with medallists in three of the four. As an Olympian himself and husband of another, Mrs Carmen Laing, in the back row, it is also appropriate that he is sitting next to another special lady in the picture.

Mrs Avril Miller represented the awardee, her late husband Dr Lennox Miller. Although not an athlete herself, she was essential in making her husband (already only the second man at the time to win two medals in the Olympic 100 metres and the only Jamaican medallist at two successive Games, in 1968 and 1972) part of the only father–daughter combination to win Olympic medals in the sport. Their daughter, Inger Miller, was a member of the US gold-medal-winning 4 × 100-metre relay team at the 1996 Atlanta Olympics.

Asafa Powell, a 2004 Olympian, sitting beside Mrs Miller, also has an Olympic family connection in that his brother Donovan Powell also represented Jamaica in the "family" event, the 100 metres, at the Sydney Olympics. At Athens, Asafa became only the second Jamaican after Don Quarrie it to make to the 100-metre and 200-metre finals at the same Games – fifth in the 100 metres, did not start in the 200 metres. Despite his series of sub-10-second clocking in 2004, Asafa still has a way to go, though, in order to match or pass Lennox Miller as Jamaica's best performer in the event at the Games.

Finally, sitting at the end, at right, is awardee Keith Gardner, to whom we have already referred. He, too, ran the Olympic 100 metres at his first Games in 1956, as well as the 110-metre hurdles and was also on the 4 × 400-metre relay team which finished fifth before being disqualified. This enabled Jamaica or the British West Indies to garner medals in this event or to reach the final in their first five Games of entry – 1948, 1952, 1956, 1960 and 1964.

Acknowledgements

The original version of this article was published in *Track and Field Jamaica: Quarterly Magazine of Jamaica's Athletics*, January–March 2006.

CHAPTER 8

A Jamaican Pioneer

Cynthia Thompson's Story

VILMA CHARLTON

As we continue to search for answers to the age-old question of why it is that Jamaicans run so fast, let us not forget Jamaica's first sprint queen, Dr Cynthia Thompson. She was an early advocate of female Jamaican athletics from as far back as the 1940s.

Cynthia was born in St Andrew, Jamaica, on November 29, 1922, and lived in the Hagley Park area for most of her early years. Interestingly, her mother was born in Trelawny, Jamaica, the area from which many Olympians have emerged or to which they have links. Her father was born in Kingston, Jamaica.

Dr Cynthia Thompson was the first Jamaican female athlete to break world track records, even though the periods were brief.

She finished sixth in the 100 metres at the 1948 Olympics in London and is Jamaica's oldest living Olympian. She recalls with bemusement her fourteen-day journey to London by banana boat and how she suffered severe seasickness, which made her lose weight and affected her physical condition for competing at the Games. Despite the long and wearying journey, she was still able to reach the 100-metre final and she broke the Olympic record with a time of 25.6 seconds in her 200-metre heat. The 200-metre race was being contested for the first time at the Olympics, therefore the Olympic record was established in a previous heat. Her teammates also performed satisfactorily. They were Mavis Evelyn in the hurdles, Carmen Phipps in the high jump, Kathleen Russell in the high jump and hurdles, and Vinton Beckett in the high jump.

Cynthia was a multiple medallist at the Central American and Caribbean (CAC) Games in 1946 and 1950. In Barranquilla, Colombia, in 1946, she won the 100 metres in a CAC record of 12.1 seconds and also won silver in the 50 metres. Four years later in

Guatemala City, she won silver in the 50 metres and 100 metres.

How did Cynthia get started in track and field? Beaming with joy while chatting about her athletic career, she excitedly related how she was introduced to a sport which became her life. Fortunately, Cynthia is blessed with a good memory, as she sadly remarked that in those days she really had not felt the urge to keep a scrapbook. The only item she can boast about keeping is her running spikes used in the 1948 Olympic Games.

It was Cynthia's schoolmate Vinton Beckett of St Hugh's High School who introduced her to track and field. At that time she was twenty-three years of age and was working at Benjamin's Manufacturing Establishment on East Street, in Kingston, Jamaica. The governing body for track and field, Vinton said, was looking for persons to represent Jamaica at the Central American and Caribbean Games. Because Cynthia was accustomed to winning every race that she had entered in high school, and because female athletes were few in number, it was easy for her to be selected.

At Cynthia's first international event in Barranquilla, she remembers competing with some very fine and fast athletes. Cynthia reiterated, "They were fast, fast, fast." For her, it was a frightening experience. She was twenty-four years old by then.

Training for her was fun. However, it soon became more serious but still enjoyable, as she claimed, in those days, there was nothing scientific about training. Cynthia would ride a bicycle to work and after work ride to Caxton Park (later George VI Memorial Park, and now National Heroes Circle) to be coached by Gerald Claude Eugene Foster, who himself was a Wolmerian athlete. She soon had to abandon riding, however, and take the tram or bus instead, as she was warned that cycling could cause injuries.

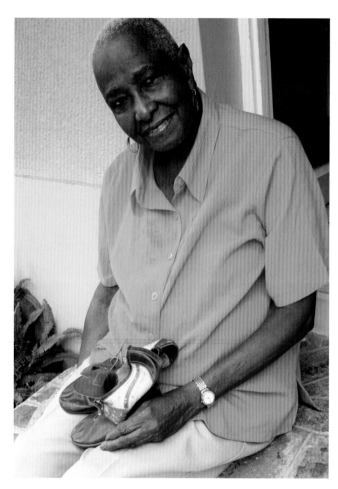

PLATE 8.1 Dr Cynthia Thompson with the shoes she competed in during the 1940s. She set an Olympic record of 25.6 seconds in the 200-metre heats at the 1948 Olympics.

Cynthia always looked forward to a special treat after training. On her way home, she got off the tram in Half Way Tree to buy her "Slim Jim" at Dairy Farmers, after which she would walk home to Hagley Park Road. The drink was a mixture made of a pint of milk, poured into a tall, fancy glass, with fruit and nuts and her favourite ice cream, a concoction she enjoys to this day.

Winning in those early years meant little to Cynthia, as running and winning for her was done only for fun. There was just no pressure, she said. No real emphasis was put on winning. All she can remember was the great fun she had, but perhaps more important to her was the socializing and the camaraderie with her training partners, teammates and coaches over the years.

This was evident when Cynthia became a Tigerbelle at Tennessee State University. She was now twenty-nine years old. It was in the early 1950s – in fact, in September 1951 – that Cynthia left Jamaica to go to Chicago Roosevelt College to further her studies. As fate would have it, one Mr W. Taffe, a popular *Gleaner* sports writer, contacted President Davis, of Tennessee State University, about Cynthia Thompson. The rest is history, as Cynthia gained a track scholarship. She represented the Tigerbelles at this university in the 100 metres, 200 metres, 4 × 100-metre relay, long jump and the 60 metres at indoor and outdoor meets.

She later moved on to study medicine at Mehary Medical College. Cynthia left Jamaica as a pharmacist, and while attending Tennessee State University she was influenced by other Jamaicans studying at Mehary.

Although she recalled her college years as being full of enjoyment, she often missed home, and, being an adult in college, she tended to stay by herself as the other students were younger. Calling herself a loner, she says she enjoys her own company at times.

After graduating from medical school, Dr Cynthia Thompson returned to Jamaica in 1966 and worked at the Bustamante Hospital for Children and later went into private practice. In track and field she made her contribution in the area of officiating as a track judge for many years.

When asked whether she would encourage youngsters to get involved in a sport and if so why, she whole-heartedly affirmed that involvement in sports keeps one healthy, and keeps youngsters out of mischief.

Cynthia had no real idol or role model, and although she had admired Hon. Arthur Wint, she claimed that she inspired herself. After all, she was the fastest female around. In her own words, "I am a go-getter."

And what kind of diet did Cynthia enjoy back then? Her diet in those days was just regular Jamaican dishes such as rice and peas, chicken and callaloo. "Definitely no fast foods," she chimed, and, of course, in her early years, that Slim Jim from Dairy Farmers was a must. Today, her favourite dishes include jerk pork and chicken.

A lover of nature, she enjoys gardening, sewing and listening to classical music, and at the age of eighty-seven years, Cynthia still drives a stylish, new Suzuki Swift motor car. Younger Olympians enjoy her company, and from time to time they ensure her involvement in many spirited or sporting activities.

Dr Cynthia Thompson was inducted into the Jamaica Amateur Athletic Association/Victoria Mutual Building Society (JAAA/VMBS) Hall of Fame on June 18, 1998. She joined the surviving members of the 1952 Helsinki Olympics gold-medal-winning 4 × 400-metre relay team (George Rhoden, Arthur Wint, Herb McKenley [now deceased], Les Laing and Byron La Beach) at the inaugural awards ceremony, held at the Jamaica Pegasus Hotel. Dr Arthur Wint was also awarded posthumously. She was honoured as Jamaica's first female finalist in an event at the Olympics. In 2000, she was also inducted in the Hall of Fame of Tennessee State University, the home of the Tigerbelles.

Thank you, Cynthia, for serving us so well as our Jamaican pioneer in track and field.

Usain Bolt

Phenomenal Track and Field Athlete

R A C H A E L   I R V I N G

When you are inspired by some great purpose, some extraordinary project, all your thoughts break their bounds. Your mind transcends limitations, your consciousness expands in every direction, and you find yourself in a new, great and wonderful world.

– The Yoga Sutras of Patanjali

Usain Bolt was born on 21 August 1986 in the rural district of Sherwood Content in Trelawny, Jamaica. He attended Waldensia Primary and All-Age School and ran in local competitions. By age twelve years, he was the fastest boy in his school. Dr Paul Auden, one of his early mentors, said that young Bolt had an in-built mechanism that would prompt him as to what time he was doing over a particular distance. From an early age, Usain was his own stopwatch.

Although Usain showed the potential to be a good sprinter, his focus was on street cricket and football. He had a boyhood dream of being a great West Indian cricketer, and by puberty his speed on the pitch was remarkable. He entered William Knibb Memorial High School at about thirteen years of age and continued focusing on cricket. The cricket coach noticed his extraordinary speed on the pitch and recommended that he try track and field events. Pablo McNeil, a 1964 and 1968 Olympian who competed in the 100 metres, became Usain's early track-and-field coach.

Usain won his first high school championship medal in 2001, placing second in the 200 metres in 22.04 seconds. However, his first appearance on the world stage at the 2001 IAAF World Youth Championships was disappointing, as he failed to qualify for the 200-metre final. By 2002 young Bolt had won both the 200- and 400-metre races at the annual Boys' and Girls' High

School Championships. This prepared him well. Later that year, Usain ignited the crowd at the IAAF World Junior Championships held in Kingston, Jamaica, when he became the youngest ever male junior champion in the 200 metres. He crossed the finish line in a time of 20.61 seconds. During his final high school championship meet in 2003, he started his multiple record-breaking trend by setting new times of 20.23 and 45.30 seconds in the 200 and 400 metres, respectively. Bolt won many more gold medals at the junior level but failed to perform to expectations in major senior games. The very Jamaicans who praised him became harsh critics.

In 2004 at the Carifta games in Bermuda, Usain ran 19.93 seconds in the 200 metres, breaking the world junior record set by Roy Martin and becoming the first teenager to run under 20 seconds in the 200 metres. In 2004, under the guidance of Fitz Coleman, Usain Bolt became a professional athlete. He was chosen as part of the Jamaican team to the 2004 Olympics but was eliminated in the preliminary rounds of the 200 metres. Usain was devastated after the elimination.

In 2005, the renowned coach Glen Mills, who had previously coached Olympian and 200 metres national record holder Donald Quarrie, stepped in. In 2005 at the World Championships in Helsinki, Finland, Usian made it to the final in the 200 metres.

At the 2006 Grand Prix in Switzerland, Usain did 19.93 seconds to finish third in the 200 metres behind Xavier Carter and Tyson Gay. He had joined the array of elite sprinters. He would now share the podium with them, standing in the bronze slot. How long would it take him to stand in the slot reserved for the gold medal winner?

In 2007, Usain set a new national record of 19.75 seconds for the 200 metres at the Jamaica National Championships. He had surpassed the old record of 19.86 seconds set by Donald Quarrie in 1971.

Usain wanted a strike at the 100 metres and kept asking his coach to let him have a go at it. Eventually, Glen Mills gave in and additional preparation was started for the 100 metres. In May 2008, at an invitational meet in Kingston, Jamaica, Usain did 9.76 seconds for the 100 metres. This was the second fastest time in the world then, surpassed only by fellow Jamaican Asafa Powell. Jamaica now had the two fastest men in the world. Later in the month, on 31 May 2008 at the Reebok Grand Prix in New York, Usain did a stupendous 9.72 seconds, smashing the world record of 9.74 seconds set by his countryman Asafa Powell.

The world was now ready for another Jesse Owens. However, the world had become numbed by the constant drug cheats in athletics. Marion Jones, America's darling of track and field, had just been implicated in the Bay Area Laboratory Co-operative (BALCO) scam. Earlier, Justin Gatlin was banned for using drugs. Could a Jamaican revitalize track and field?

Bio-statisticians using data collected over a span of one hundred years predicted that a time of 9.69 seconds in the 100 metres would not be reached before the year 2030. In the 100-metre final at the 2008 Olympics, Usain, alias "Lightning", did 9.69 seconds; he slowed down to celebrate before the end of the race, and had been discombobulated by a loose shoelace during the race. His coach, Glen Mills, said Usain could have done 9.52 seconds. A corollary of a study called "How Fast Could Usain Bolt Have Run? A Dynamical Study" concluded that 9.5 seconds is well within the reach of Usain Bolt in the near future (Eriksen et al. 2008). Michael Johnson postulated that his world record of 19.32 seconds for the 200 metres would remain intact after the 2008 Olympics. He underesti-

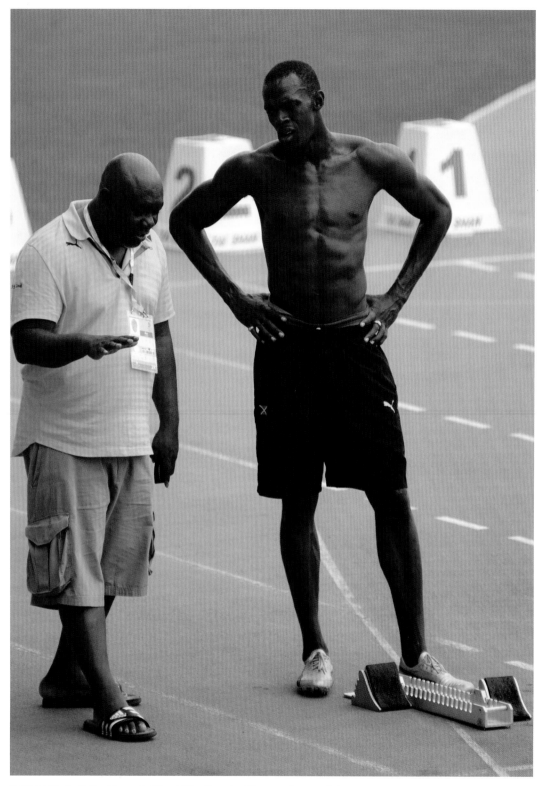

PLATE 9.1 Usain Bolt with coach Glen Mills. (*Jamaica Observer* photograph.)

mated this phenomenal Jamaican. As the world stood in amazement, Johnson's record fell. Usain smashed the record and set a new world record of 19.30 seconds. By his remarkable display on the track he nullified the theory of sprint prowess and its link to body types. Most sprinters are below 6 feet 3 inches in height. "Lightning" is a towering 6 feet 5 inches. Usain, aided by Nesta Carter, Michael Frater and Asafa Powell, went on to set another world record in the 4 × 100-metre relay. Usain became the first man since Carl Lewis to win 100-, 200- and 4 × 100-metre races at a single Olympics and the first in the history of the Games to set three world records in track-and-field events in a single year.

Life after the 2008 Olympic Games

On Sunday 17 May 2009, just two weeks after crashing his BMW motor car in Jamaica and having minor surgery on his feet, Usain Bolt did 14.35 seconds in Manchester, England, to set an unofficial world record for the 150 metres. Usain continued running for an additional 50 metres after the finish line (http://www. sportsillustrated.cnn.com). On Thursday, 11 June 2009, three weeks after setting a new world record for the 150 metres in England, Usain competed in the Festival of Excellence meet in Toronto, Canada, and cruised past his competitors in the 100 metres in a time of 10.00 seconds (http://www.cbc.ca). He said after the race, "Some days you have good days and some days you have bad days, I guess you can put this down as a bad day for me." The previous day he had been named Laureus World Sportsman of the Year. He was awarded for his historical performance at the 2008 Olympics in Beijing. Edwin Moses, chairman of Laureus Academy, and

Michael Johnson, Academy member and holder of the 200-metre world record prior to it being broken, presented the award to Usain in Toronto (http://www. sports.espn.go.com).

Scientists from the Institute of Theoretical Astrophysics, University of Oslo, Norway, had concluded after his phenomenal run in the 2008 Beijing Olympics that 9.5 seconds in the 100 metres was reachable by him in the near future (Eriksen et al. 2008). At the World Championships in August 2009 he lowered his own 100-metre world record by 0.11 seconds.

For forty years prior to Usain, records fell by a hundredth of a second at a time. When a group of scientists commissioned by the IAAF carried out the biomechanical analysis of the 100-metre race, it was shown that by 20 metres into the race Usain, was ahead of his competitors and for each 20-metre interval he got further away, reaching a top speed of 27.45 miles per hour at the 65-metre mark. From 80 to 100 metres Usain slowed down considerably, by then he was far ahead of the other finalists. His time for the last 20 metres is 0.05 seconds slower than his fastest 20-metre split of 1.61 seconds (http://www.berlin.iaaf.org). Tyson Gay, who collected the silver medal for that race, gave the race his all. Tyson set an American record of 9.71 seconds but was unable to keep up with "Lightning" Bolt. Can Usain go much faster in the near future? Many pundits are predicting Usain Bolt to set a world record time of 9.40 seconds in the 100 metres.

Usain also took command of the 200-metre final at the twelfth IAAF World Championships and did a stunning 19.19 seconds to smash his previous world record of 19.30 seconds. Later in the championships, he took another gold in the 4 × 100 metres. His relay team, which included Asafa Powell, Michael Frater and Steve Mullings, set a championship record. To immortalize

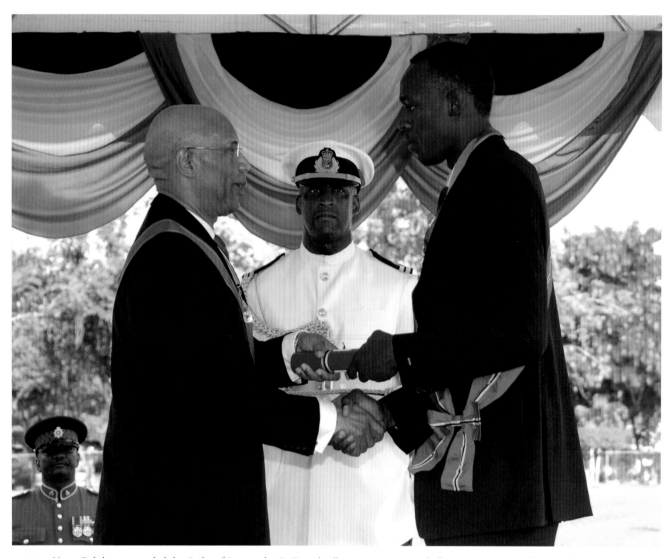

PLATE 9.2 Usain Bolt being awarded the Order of Jamaica by Sir Patrick Allen, governor general of Jamaica. (*Jamaica Observer* photograph.)

his feats in Berlin, Usain was given a piece of the Berlin Wall.

On Sunday, 13 September 2009, Usain brought the curtain down at the World Athletics finals with a smashing 19.68 seconds for the 200 metres. Bolt was earmarked for China's Shanghai International meet on 20 September and the Daegu Pre-Championship meet in South Korea on 25 September 2009, but his managers advised the organizing committees that he was too tired to compete.

Usain returned to Jamaica on 14 September 2009, where he was welcomed by government officials at a press conference at Terra Nova Hotel in Kingston. The following day, the prime minister of Jamaica announced that Usain Bolt was to be awarded the Order of Jamaica, the nation's fourth highest order. Usain was also designated ambassador-at-large and will enjoy diplomatic status wherever he travels, and a highway in Jamaica was renamed the Usain Bolt Highway (http://www.jamaica-gleaner.com) in his honour.

Usain Bolt is representative of "Brand Jamaica" athleticism. The question of whether his sprinting prowess is inherited or nurtured will be debated for a long time. His father, Wellesley Bolt, has implied that eating yams may have played a role in his prowess. From a scientific standpoint, a study conducted by Irving et al. (2009), based on scientific analysis of DNA samples, has determined that most Jamaicans are of West African ancestry and have the genes that predispose them to be good sprinters. Vilma Charlton, lecturer in physical education and herself an Olympian, has alluded to the positive effects of physical conditioning gained through a good physical education in school programme. Irving et al. (2009) continue to study Jamaican athletes, considering the psychological and neurological components associated with sustained elite performance. The researchers have found empirical evidence linking sustained speed to control of emotion and regulation of serotonin levels (unpublished data).

Whether nature or nurture, Usain is a phenomenal athlete and a remarkable ambassador for Jamaica.

References

Eriksen, H.K., J.R. Kristiansen, O. Langangen and I.K. Wehis. 2008. Velocity dispersions in a cluster of stars: How fast could Usain Bolt have run? A dynamical study. American Journal of Physics 77 (3): 224–28.

Irving, R., R. Scott, L. Irwin, E. Morrison, V. Charlton, A. Austin, S. Headley, F. Kolkhorst and Y. Pitsiladis. 2009. The ACTN3 R577X polymorphism in elite Jamaican and US sprinters. *Medicine and Science in Sports and Exercise* 41 (5): 165.

Scott, R., R. Irving, L. Irwin, M. Morrison, V. Charlton, K. Austin, D. Tladi, A. Headley, F. Kolkhorst, N. Yang, K. North and Y.P. Pitsiladis. 2010. ACTN3 and ACE genotypes in elite Jamaican and US sprinters. *Medicine and Science in Sports and Exercise* 42 (1): 107–15.

CHAPTER 10

Melaine Walker

Olympic Games and World Championships Gold-Medal Hurdler

RACHAEL IRVING

For someone who does not like the 400-metre hurdles, Melaine has done extremely well. She won the Olympic gold in Beijing in 2008, in a record time of 52.64 seconds, and declared immediately afterward, "I absolutely hated it." She hated it but she executed the race with complete finesse. She ran conservatively in the early part of the race and then accelerated past Sheena Tosta of the United States to take the coveted gold. Based on her performance at the 2008 Olympic Games, she was named Jamaica's sportswoman of the year jointly with Veronica Campbell-Brown, who won the 200-metre gold at the 2008 Olympics. A year later, in 2009, at the twelfth IAAF World Championships in Athletics in Berlin, Melaine demolished America's Lashinda Demus to take the gold medal in a championship record time of 52.42 seconds. Melaine became the second fastest women in the world over the 400-metre hurdles, superseded only by Russian Yuliya Pechonkina with a time of 52.34 seconds.

Melaine is the second Jamaican woman to win gold and set an Olympic record in the 400-metre hurdles (Deon Hemmings was the first, in 1996). Melaine, however, carved her name in Jamaica's annals by being the first Jamaican woman to win Olympic Games and World Championships gold medals in the 400-metre hurdles. She believes perseverance accounts for her success. In 1999 with a broken arm, Melaine did 11.63 and 23.75 seconds in the 100 and 200 metres, respectively, to defeat Veronica Campbell. Melaine competing in class two then also did 13.52 seconds to take gold in the 100-metre hurdles. She was surprised that she had won three gold medals in a single year at the high school championships. She won bronze at the 2000 World Junior Championships in Santiago, Chile; silver at the 2002 World Junior Championships in Kingston, Jamaica; and bronze at the 2007 World Athletics final in Stuttgart, Germany.

Who Is Melaine Walker?

Melaine was born on 1 January 1983 in Kingston, Jamaica. She started track and field just for fun at three years of age. She attended St Jago High School and received a track scholarship to Essex County College. She later transferred to the University of Texas at Austin. Melaine was a NCAA track-and-field South Central Region honouree at university, and she graduated with a Bachelor of Science degree in early childhood education. Melaine trains with the renowned Stephen Francis of Maximizing Velocity and Power (MVP) Track Club in Jamaica. Stephen has nurtured former world record holder Asafa Powell, 100-metre Olympic Games and World Championships gold medallist Shelly-Ann Fraser, and World Championships 100-metre gold medal hurdler Brigitte Foster-Hylton. Melaine had wanted to switch back to the 100-metre hurdles, but Stephen felt she was better at the 400 metres.

Melaine is strong on family. Her mother is always around her. Although she grew up in the inner-city area of Maxfield Avenue in Kingston, her parents expected her to do well. She was expected to follow her brothers and sisters who had done well. She tries her best not to let her parents down.

Melaine had no confidence in herself while growing up. Her father, however, always believed in her ability. He remarked on a television programme that, just before her win in Berlin, he went to shave his face because it did not look like the face of the father of a 400-metre hurdles world champion.

Reflecting on track and field, Melaine said, "It helped me to be more confident; I was shy." Melaine confesses to now loving the cameras and public speaking. She encourages youngsters to get involved in sports, as it helps them not to be idle.

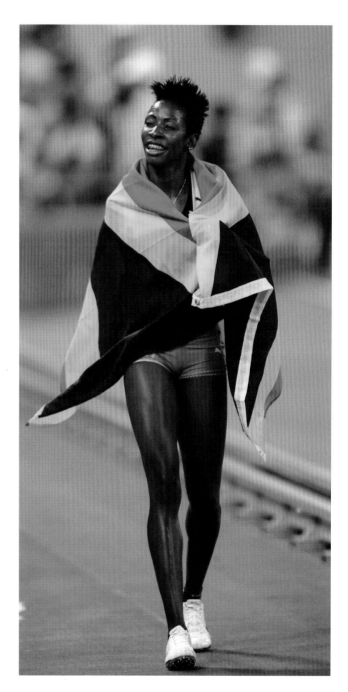

PLATE 10.1 Melaine Walker is the second Jamaican woman to win Olympic gold and set an Olympic record in the 400-metre hurdles. (*Jamaica Observer* photograph.)

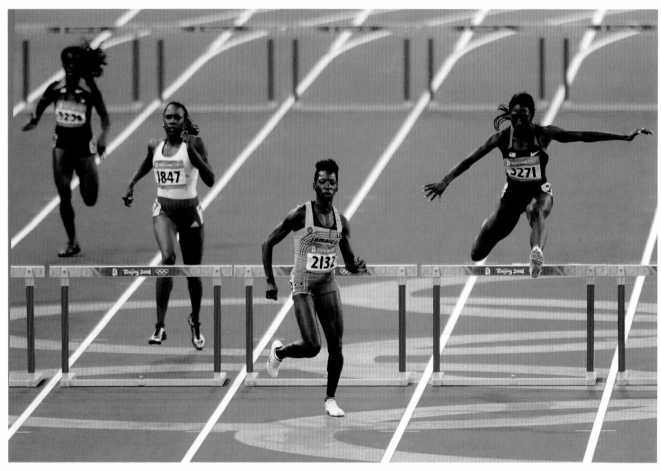

PLATE 10.2 Melaine Walker on her way to winning gold in the women's 400-metre hurdles in a time of 52.64 seconds at the 2008 Beijing Olympic Games. (*Jamaica Observer* photograph.)

Melaine was awarded the country's fifth highest honour, the Order of Distinction, Officer Class, for her contribution to track and field in Jamaica. She no longer lives in the inner city, but she visits regularly. She said she will never forget her past. She thinks that if she could rise above poverty and excel at the international level, any inner-city youth can. She loves interacting with children. At the end of her track career, she hopes to utilize her skills in early childhood education, which was her major at the University of Texas.

Acknowledgements

Information for this article was obtained from Melaine Walker and Bruce James, manager of MVP Track Club.

SECTION 3

The History of Jamaican Sprinting in Pictures

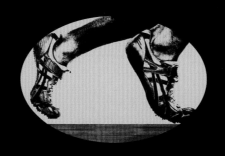

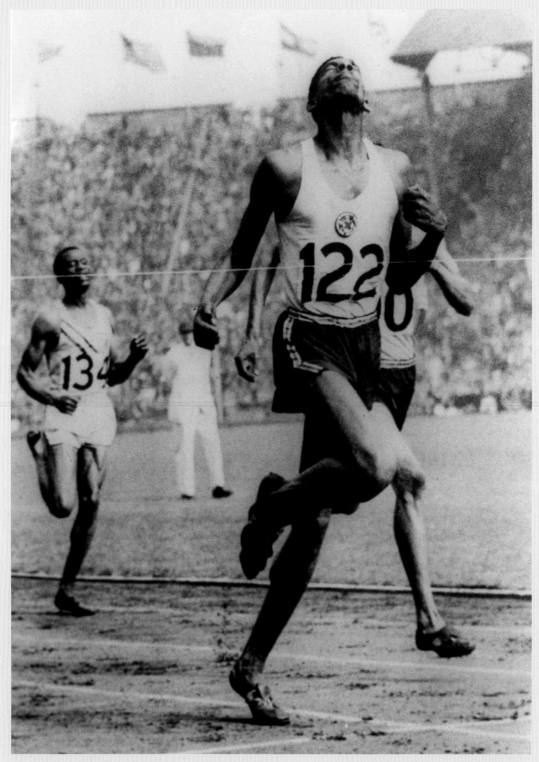

ARTHUR WINT created history by winning Jamaica's first gold in the men's 400 metres in the 1948 Olympic Games in London. This win began a tradition of excellence by Jamaican sprinters. (National Library of Jamaica photograph.)

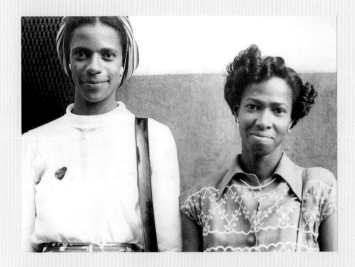

DR CYNTHIA THOMPSON (*right*) was Jamaica's first sprint queen. She placed sixth in the women's 100 metres at the 1948 Olympic Games in London. She is pictured here with Ruth Cattouse, British Honduran sprint champion. (*Gleaner* photograph.)

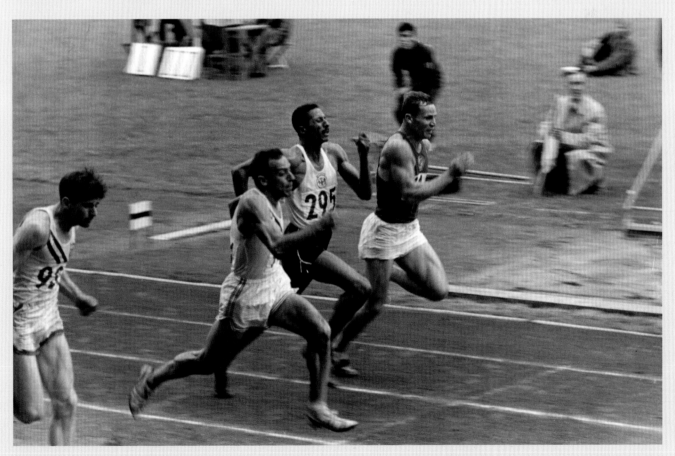

HERB MCKENLEY (*second right*) and Lindy Remigino in the epic 100-metre final at the 1952 Olympic Games in Helsinki. A photo analysis decided who got the gold: both men were hand-timed at 10.4 seconds. (National Library of Jamaica photograph.)

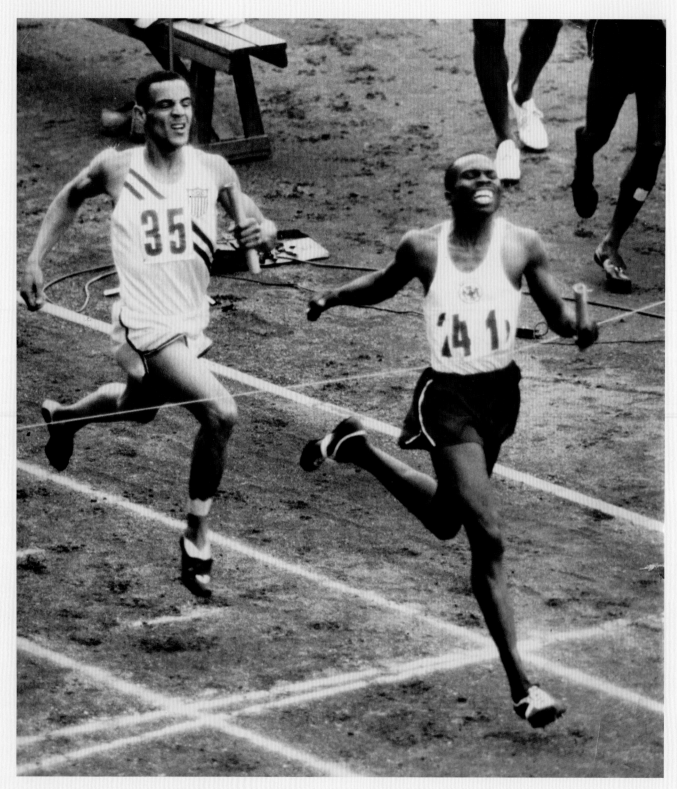

GEORGE RHODEN winning ahead of Mel Whithead in the 1952 Olympic Games in Helsinki. (National Library of Jamaica photograph.)

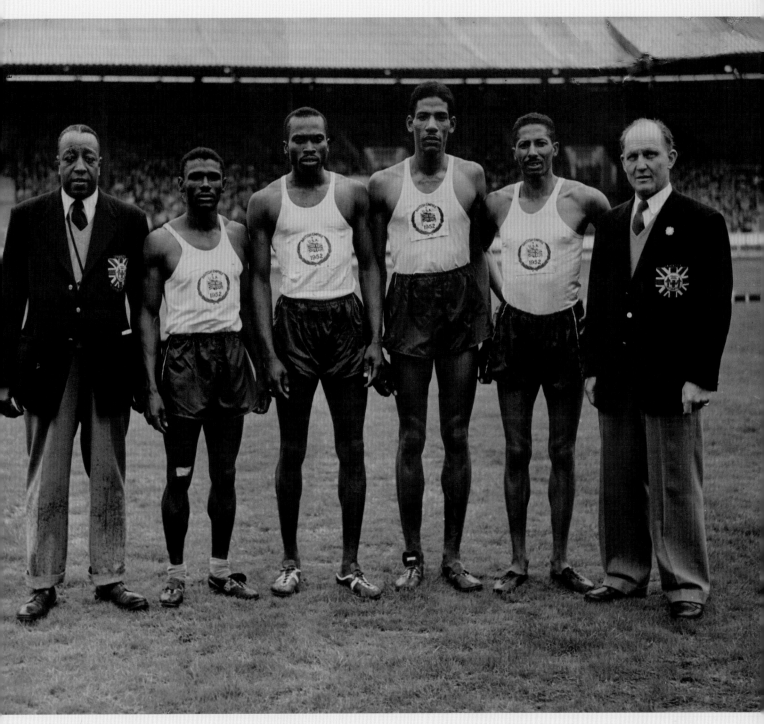

The winning 4 × 100 metre team at the 1952 Helsinki Olympic Games with their coach and manager. From left are Joe Yancey (coach), LES LAING, GEORGE RHODEN, ARTHUR WINT, HERB MCKENLEY and Sir Herbert MacDonald (manager). (National Library of Jamaica photograph.)

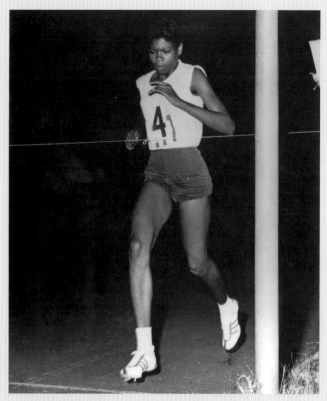

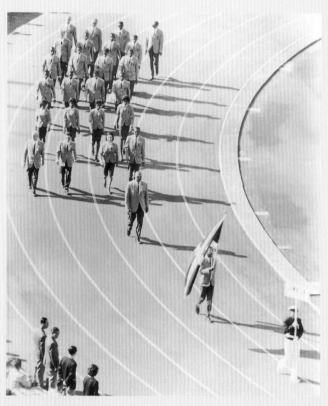

UNA MORRIS, the then-sixteen-year-old sprint sensation. She was Sportswoman of the Year in 1963 and 1964, and placed fourth in the 200-metre final in the 1964 Olympic Games. Dr Una Morris-Chong is now a radiologist in California.

The Jamaican team, led by GEORGE KERR, parading during the opening ceremony of the 1964 Olympics in Tokyo, Japan. This was the first national team of an independent Jamaica.

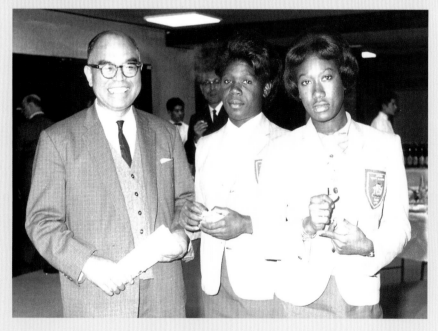

VILMA CHARLTON, three-time Olympian (1964, 1968, 1972) at centre. To the right is CARMEN SMITH-BROWN, silver medallist in the 100 metres at the 1966 Commonwealth Games in Kingston, Jamaica. Both women were members of the 4 × 100-metre gold-medal team at the 1966 Central American and Caribbean Games in San Juan, Puerto Rico. A Japanese official is at the left.

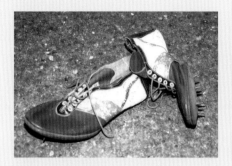 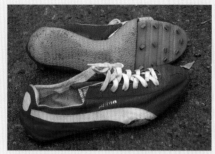 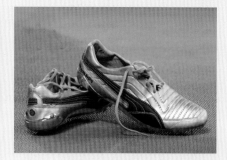

The evolution of the shoes of Jamaican champions: (*left*) 1940s–1950s, long spikes worn on dirt track by former Olympic and world record holder Dr Cynthia Thompson; (*middle*) 1960s–1970s, track shoes, worn on chevron surface by Olympian and Central America and Caribbean Games medallist Vilma Charlton and eventually banned from competitive games after the Mexico Olympic Games; (*right*) 2008, winning shoes worn by multiple world and Olympic record holder Usain Bolt.

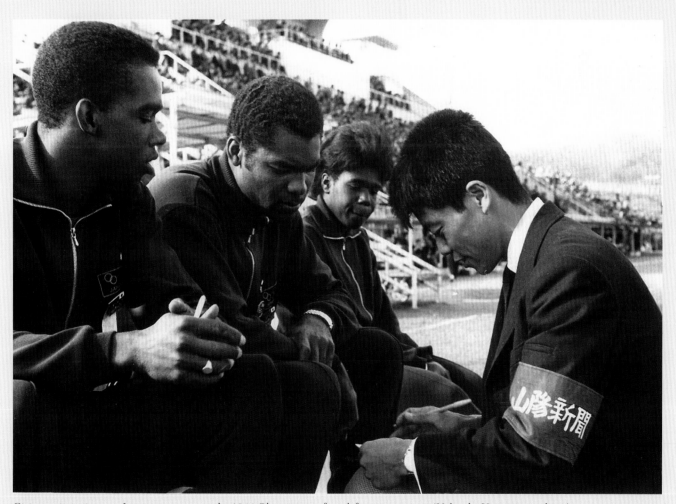

Giving an interview to a Japanese reporter at the 1964 Olympics are, from left, LINDY HEADLEY (Nebraska University graduate), DR PATRICK ROBINSON (University of the West Indies graduate) and VILMA CHARLTON (Pepperdine University graduate).

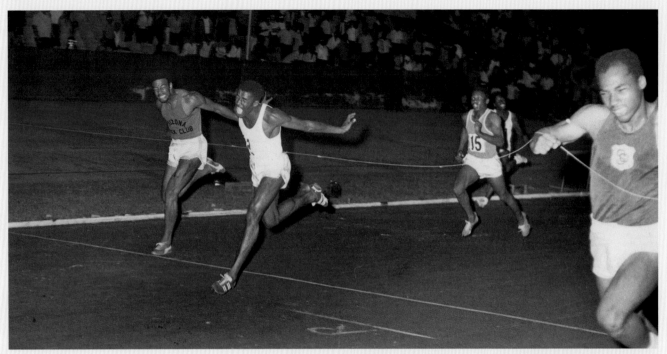

LENNOX MILLER (*far right*), representing the University of Southern California, qualified for the men's 100 metres in both the 1968 Mexico and 1972 Munich Olympic Games. He won silver in Mexico and bronze in Munich. (National Library of Jamaica photograph.)

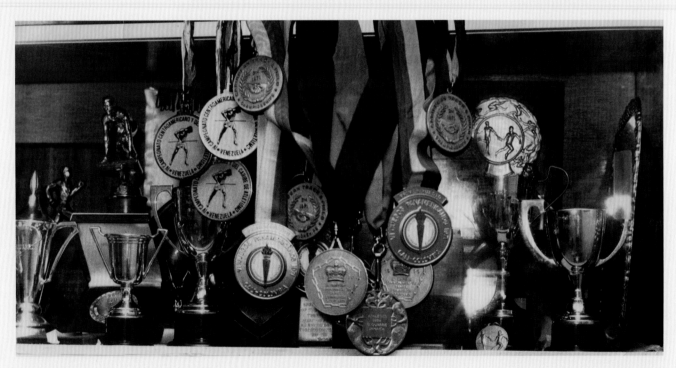

The legendary DONALD QUARRIE'S medals. He won a total of fifteen gold medals in international meets, including the men's 200 metres at the 1976 Montreal Olympic Games. (National Library of Jamaica photograph.)

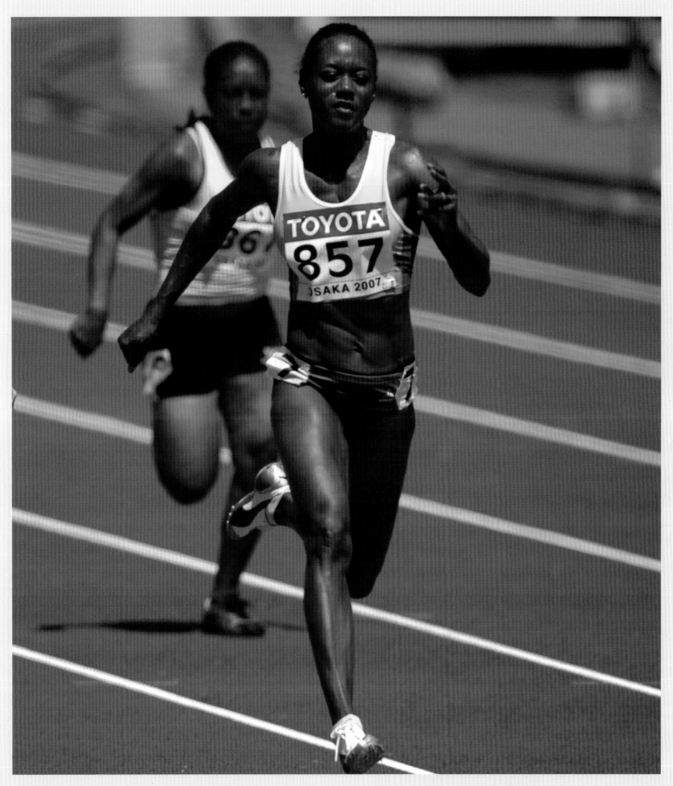

MERLENE OTTEY (*in front*) holds the record for the female athlete who has won the most medals in the Olympic Games. At fifty years old she holds the record for the oldest competitor at the European Championships. (*Jamaica Observer* photograph.)

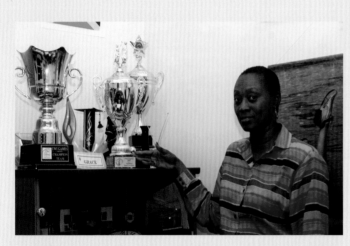

GRACE JACKSON, one of Jamaica's outstanding female athletes, won silver in the 1988 Seoul Olympic Games. She is director of sports development at the University of the West Indies, Mona, Jamaica. Here she displays medals won by the university's students. (*Gleaner* photograph.)

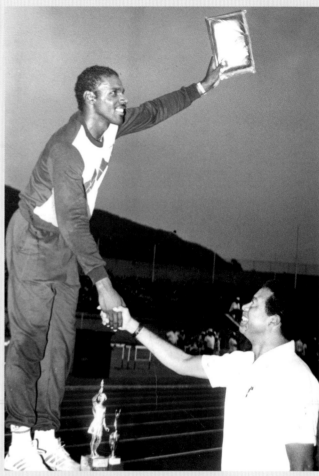

BERT CAMERON was a member of the men's 4 × 400-metre relay team that won silver in the 1988 Seoul Olympic Games. (*Gleaner* photograph.)

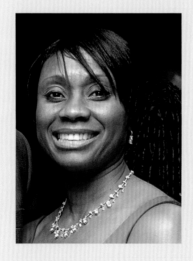

JULIET CUTHBERT was the first woman to win silver medals for Jamaica in two events at the same Olympic Games. She won silver in the 100 metres and the 200 metres at the 1992 Barcelona Olympic Games. She was a member of the women's 4 × 100-metre relay team that won bronze at the 1996 Atlanta Olympic Games. (*Gleaner* photograph.)

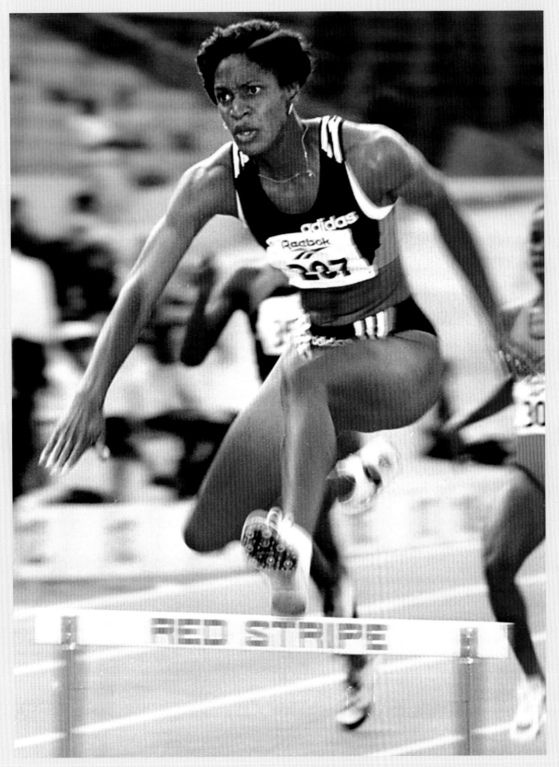

DEON HEMMINGS, the first Jamaican woman to win an Olympic gold. She won the 400-metre hurdles in 1996. (*Jamaica Observer* photograph.)

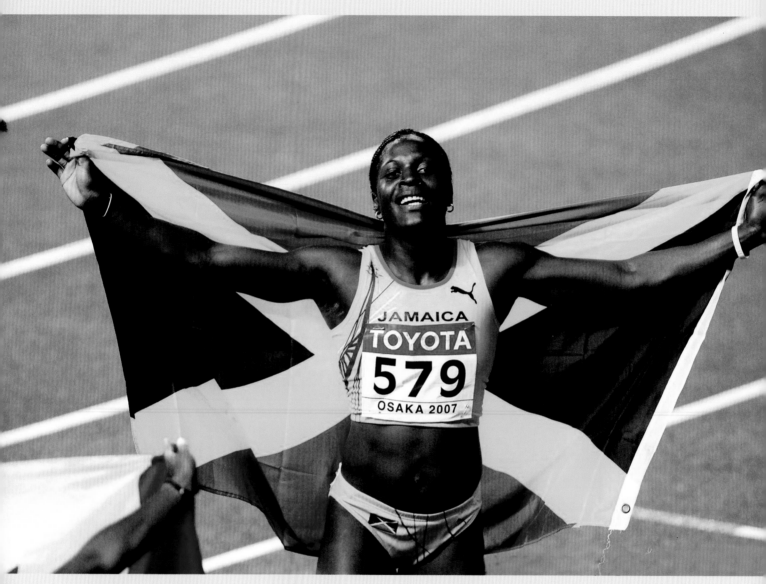

DELLOREEN ENNIS-LONDON won bronze in the women's 100-metre hurdles at the 2007 World Championships in Osaka. (*Gleaner* photograph.)

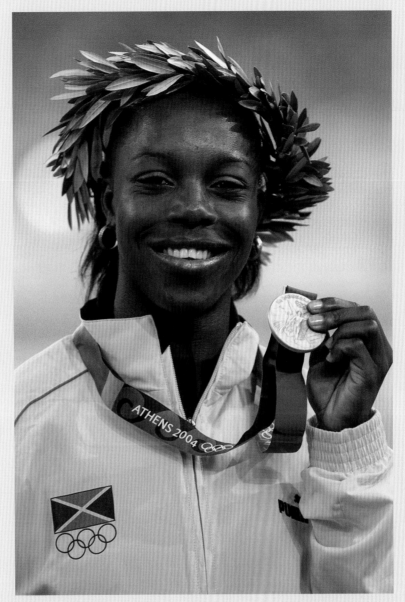

The most decorated track and field athlete in Jamaica and possibly in the world is VERONICA CAMPBELL-BROWN. She received the Order of Distinction (Commander Class) from the Government of Jamaica in 2008 for her stellar performance in athletics. Veronica has won medals at every level of international competition, from junior to senior. In fact, she could be considered the world's most decorated female athlete. To date, she is a five-time Olympic medallist (three gold, one silver, one bronze); six-time World Championship medallist (one gold, five silver); 60-metre World Champion in 2010; and second female athlete in history to win the 200 metres back-to-back at the Olympic Games (2004 and 2008).

Veronica had the benefit of being mentored by prominent role models in Jamaican society through the Grace, Kennedy Company Limited mentorship programme. In turn, she has become a role model herself: she is active in charity work, the author of *A Better You: Inspirations for Life's Journey* and, was, in 2009, appointed by the Government of Jamaica to be UNESCO ambassador of sports for peace and to promote gender equality in sports.

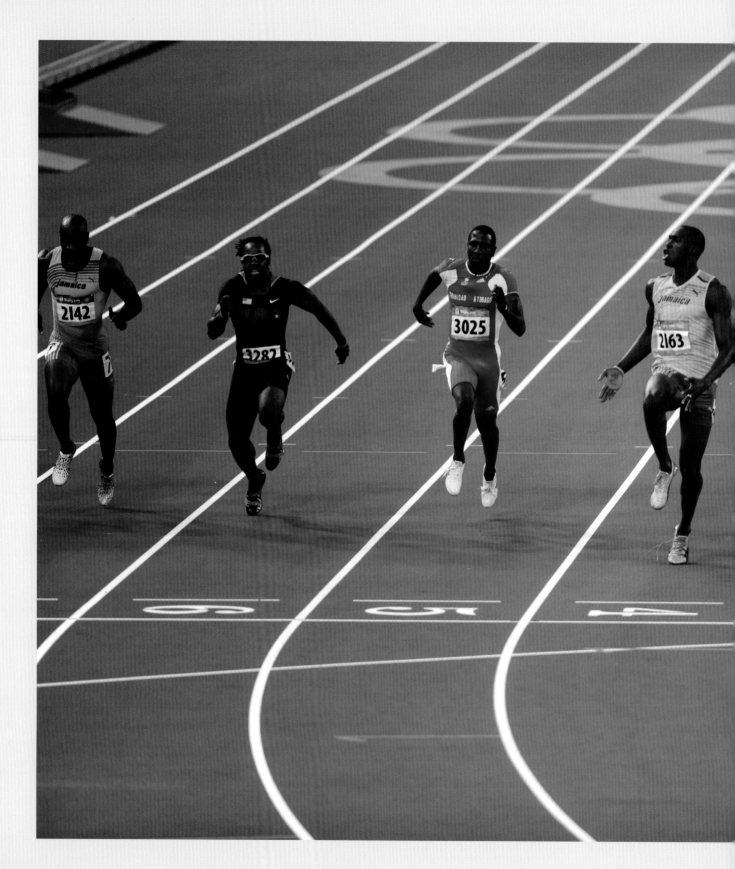

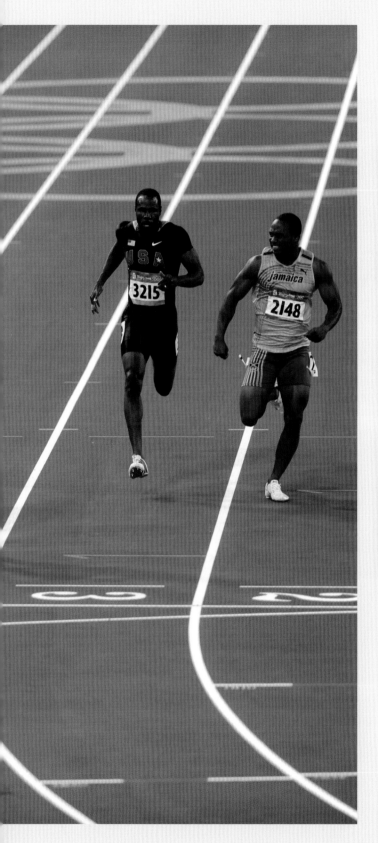

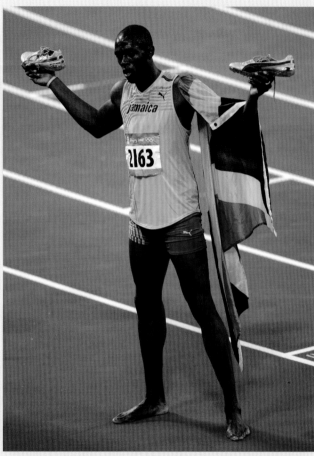

USAIN BOLT established a new world and Olympic record of 9.69 seconds (*above and centre*) men's 100 metres at the 2008 Olympic Games in Beijing. Pictured at far left is ASAFA POWELL, and at far right is MICHAEL FRATER. (*Jamaica Observer* photographs.)

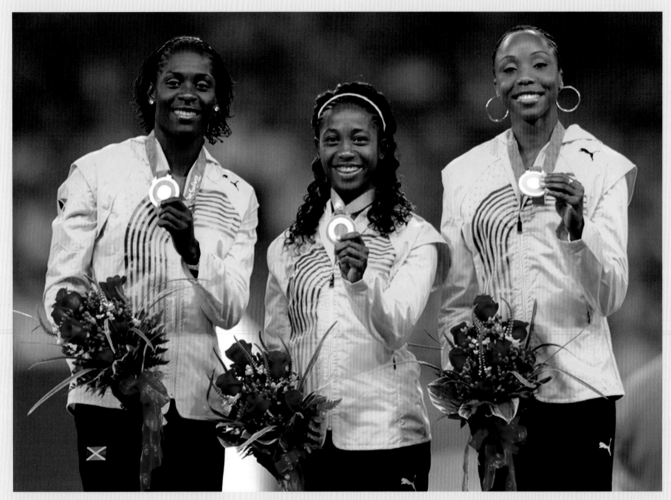

Jamaica swept all the medals in the women's 100-metre finals at the 2008 Olympic Games in a historic 1–2–2 finish. From left are KERRON STEWART (silver), SHELLY-ANN FRASER (gold) and SHERONE SIMPSON (silver). (*Jamaica Observer* photograph.)

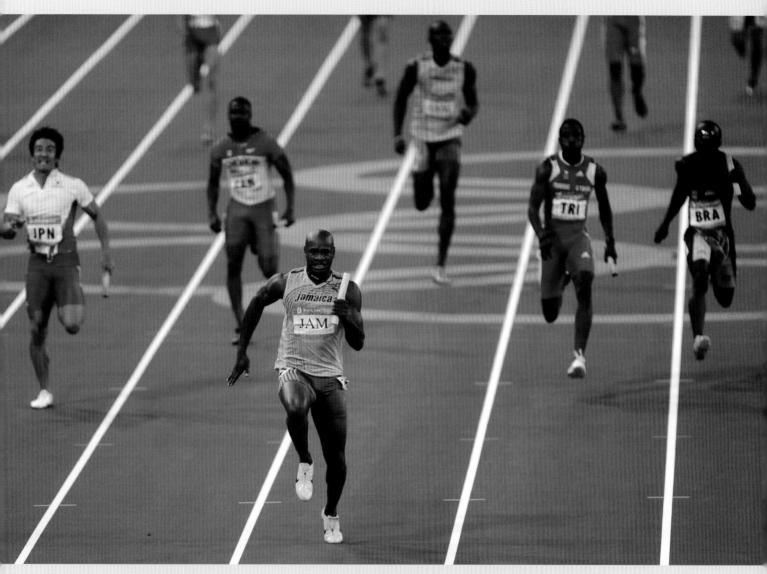

ASAFA POWELL ran a record leg in the men's 4 × 100-metre relay in the 2008 Beijing Olympic Games, a world record of 37.10 seconds was set by the team. Bolt continued running and was ahead of some of the other runners in the final leg. (*Jamaica Observer* photograph.)

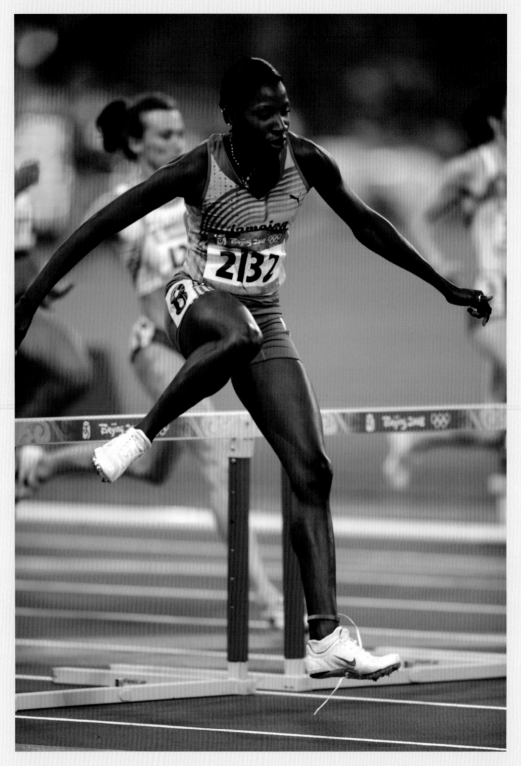

MELAINE WALKER won gold in the women's 400-metre hurdles in the 2008 Beijing Olympics in a time of 52.64 seconds. (*Jamaica Observer* photograph.)

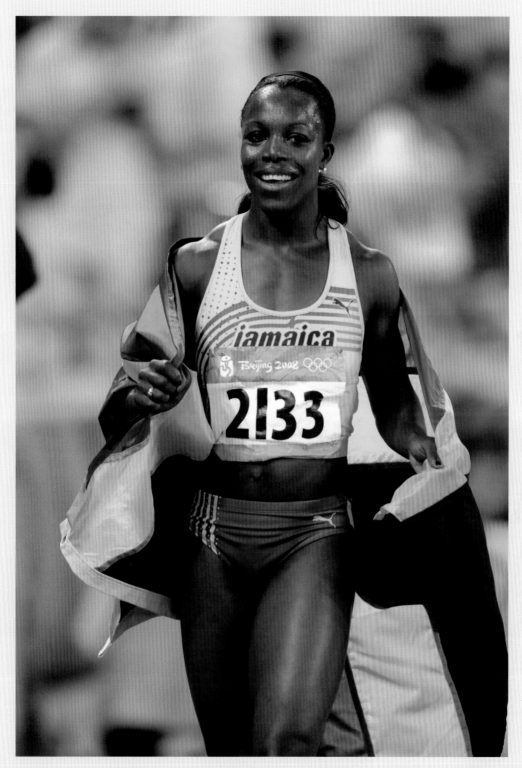

VERONICA CAMPBELL-BROWN successfully defended her 200-metre gold medal at the 2008 Beijing Olympic Games in a time of 21.74 seconds. (*Jamaica Observer* photograph.)

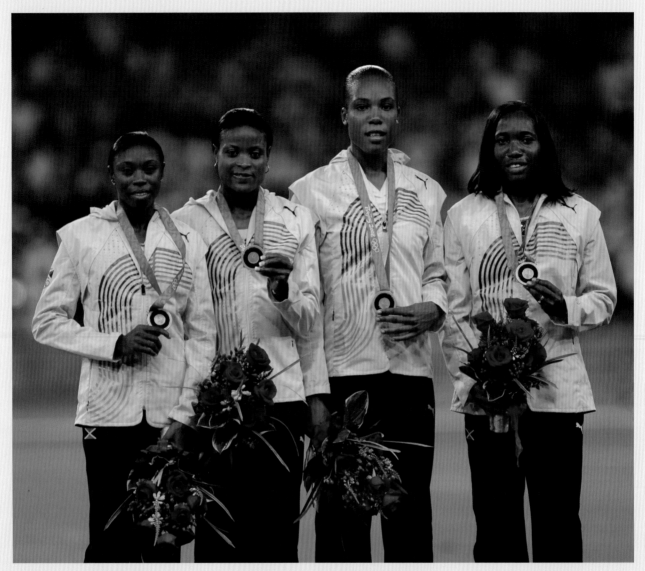

From left are SHERICKA WILLIAMS, SHEREEFA LLOYD, ROSEMARIE WHYTE and NOVLENE WILLIAMS-MILLS, winners of the bronze medal in the women's 4 × 400-metre relay at the 2008 Beijing Olympic Games. (*Jamaica Observer* photograph.)

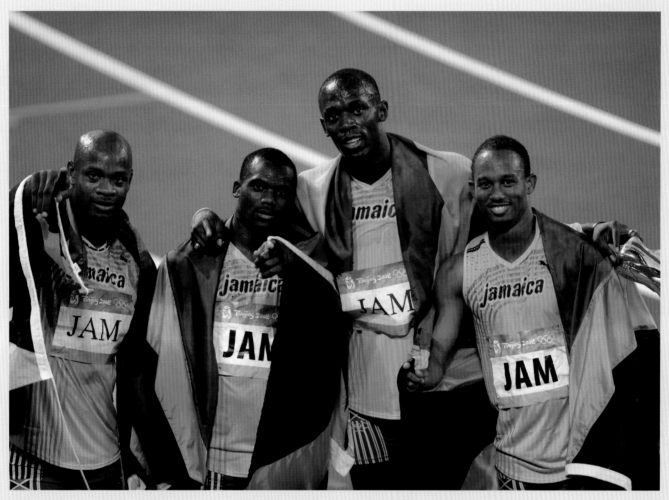

The 4 × 100-metre men's relay team set a world and Olympic record of 37.10 seconds at the 2008 Olympic Games in Beijing. From left are ASAFA POWELL, NESTER CARTER, USAIN BOLT and MICHAEL FRATER posing after their victory. (*Jamaica Observer* photograph.)

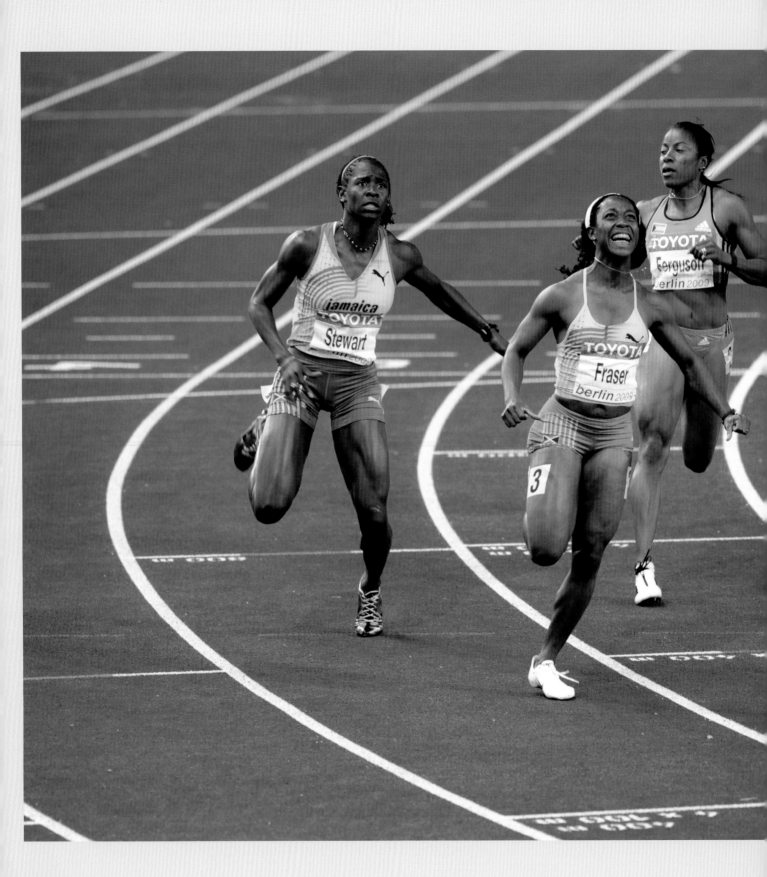

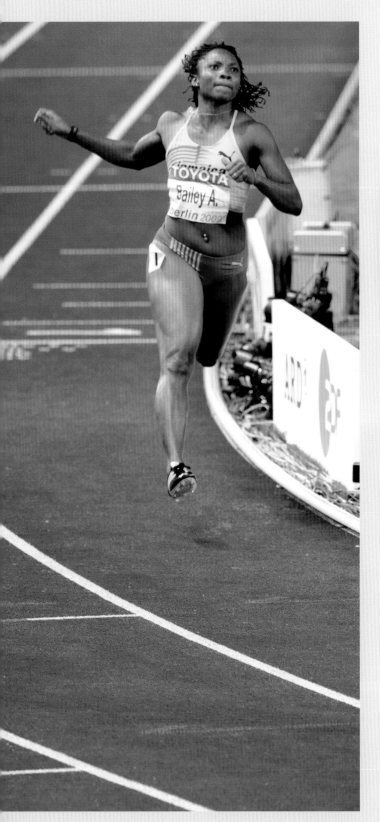

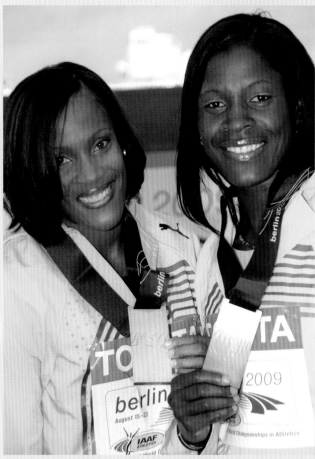

BRIGITTE FOSTER-HYLTON and DELLOREEN ENNIS-LONDON celebrating their gold and bronze medals in the women's 100-metre hurdles at the 2009 World Championships in Berlin.

SHELLY-ANN FRASER takes the gold in women's 100 metres at the 2009 Berlin World Championships. KERRON STEWART (*extreme left*) wins silver and Carmelita Jeter (United States, *not pictured*) bronze. ALEEN BAILEY (*extreme right*) gave a great performance despite the fact that she did not win a medal. (*Jamaica Observer* photograph.)

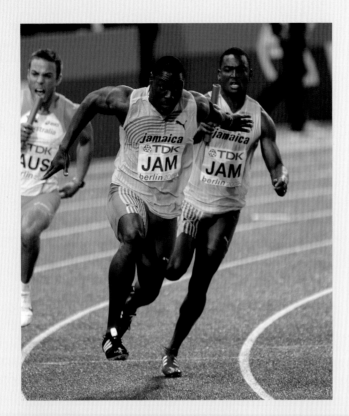

STEVE MULLINGS passes the baton to DWIGHT THOMAS in the heats for the men's 4 × 100-metre relay in the 2009 World Championships in Berlin. The team won gold in a Championship record. (*Jamaica Observer* photograph.)

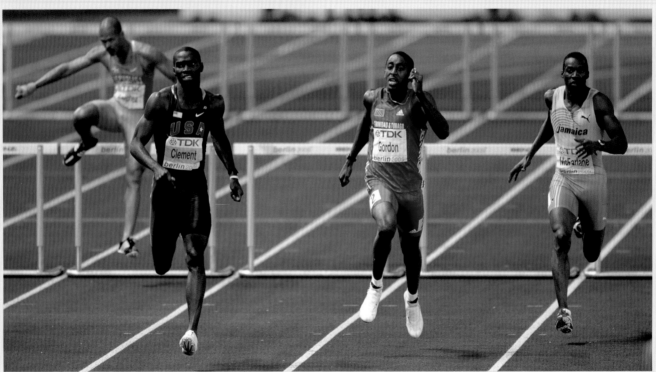

DANNY MCFARLANE (*far right*), veteran Olympian and finalist in the 400-metre hurdles at the 2009 World Championships in Berlin. (*Jamaica Observer* photograph.)

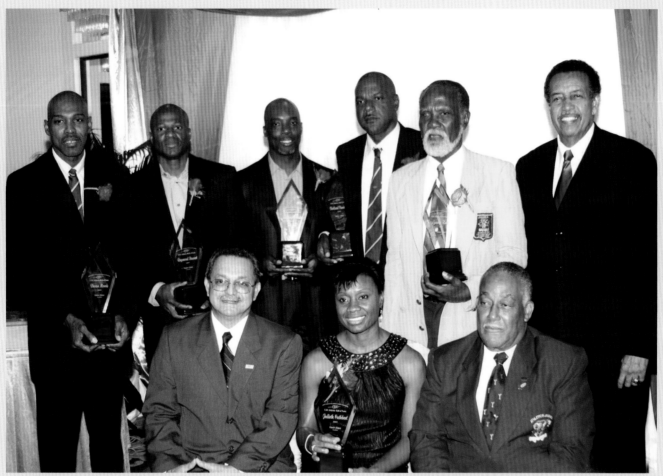

Six athletes were inducted into the Central American and Caribbean Athletics Confederation Hall of Fame in January 2008 at the Hilton Hotel in Kingston, Jamaica. Standing, from left, are Devon Morris, Raymond Stewart, Winthrop Graham, Bertland Cameron, George Kerr and Howard Aris (JAAA president). Seated, from left, are Victor Lopez (CACAC president), Juliet Cuthbert and Neville (Teddy) McCook (IAAF area representative).

SECTION 4

The Cultural Norms That Make Jamaicans Unique

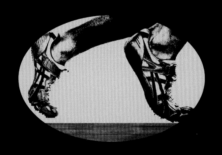

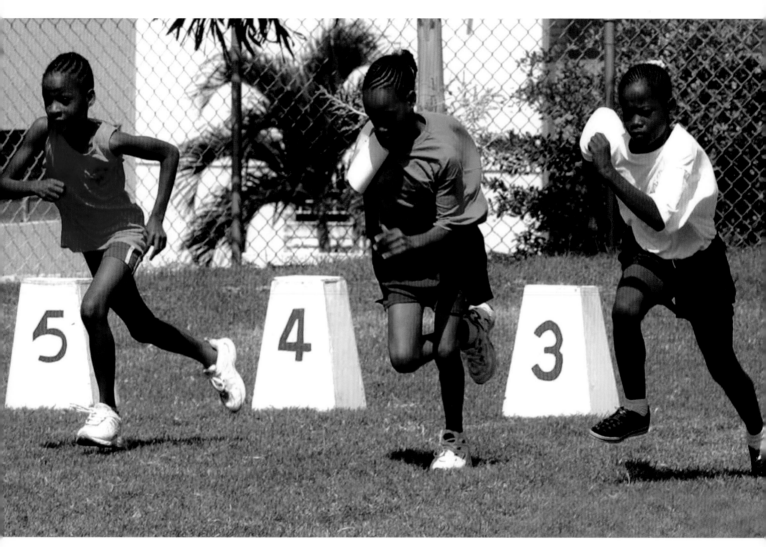

PLATE 11.1 The competitive spirit is nurtured in Jamaican children from an early age. (*Gleaner* photograph.)

CHAPTER 11

Run for Your Life

AGGREY IRONS

The movie *Cool Runnings* has successfully documented Jamaica's entry into the area of bobsledding. *Hot running* has always symbolized our traditional heroics in track and field – but still no movie. Jamaica's running heroes, such as Wint, McKenley, Ottey, Quarrie, Miller, Campbell-Brown, Powell, Bolt and company read like a veritable alphabet from A to Z, causing the rest of the world to wonder what the secret is. Well, a secret is not a secret if it is revealed, so I will not be found guilty of telling secrets – but here are a few clues.

Tradition

The first school bell rings; it is five minutes to eight; and you are eight hundred yards from school – you walk faster while conversing with your friends. The last bell rings; it's eight o'clock; you are eighty yards away from the gate – you all sprint while the bell is ringing; you make the assembly line, just in time. You grow, you develop, you learn to beat the clock – you *run* for your life.

You are a Jamaican child in rural Jamaica. Sometimes your feet are bare, sometimes you wear sneakers – the shoes formerly known as "puss boots". You stone mangoes – the farmer is coming – you *run* for your life.

You have no bat; you have no ball; no special equipment. On your marks, get set, *go* becomes your creed – you *run* for your life.

You have been naughty, Granny is coming with the switch – you *run* for your life.

You are in school; there are the Red House, Blue House, Green House teams – you *run* for your house. There is the primary, the preparatory school, the high school, the college – you *run* for your school. You are among the best, you have limited opportunities for income – you *run* for your life.

Some people around are inclined to violence, there is no "on your marks", no "get set", just a gunshot – you *run* for your life.

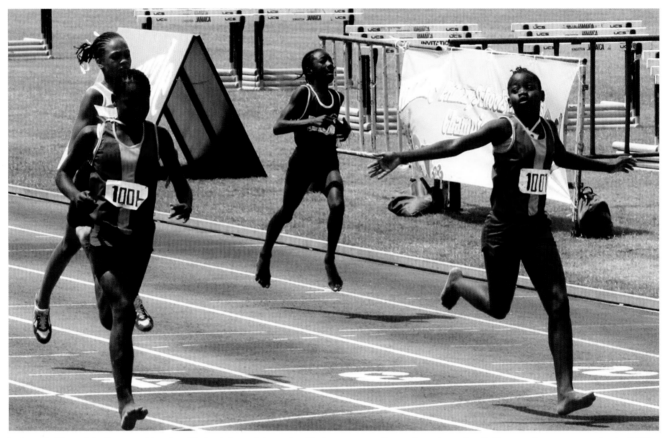

PLATE 11.2 The spirit of competition in athletics is honed through athletic meets starting at the primary level. Here students compete in the 2009 Institute of Sports/Swizzle Primary Athletic championships at the National Stadium. (*Gleaner* photograph.)

Jamaica's reputation for fast running in the post-war period has left us with the reputation of being the fastest people in the world. You live your life hearing, *good, better, best*: you never let it rest – you *run* for your life.

Individualism

Running is primarily an individual sport. Jamaican individualism makes us the most competitive people in the world. After all, "We run things, things no run we." There is room for the well behaved and the not-so-well behaved.

Life teaches us that when we have a level playing-field and we even receive our own lane – the rest is up to us. Think of a sport that proportionally and directly rewards effort and hard work – *running*. When we say "soon come", we may be late but sometimes we have to run for our lives.

Teamwork

It is fascinating that running facilitates both individualism and teamwork simultaneously but that's the kind of people we are. Because of our "out of many one people" philosophy, we are a complex gene pool of focused individuals who know the benefits of working together. We were once slaves – we have to work together and sometimes we have to run for our lives.

Rhythm and Reggae

The only activity that we do better than running is singing and dancing. When we put that rhythm into our sprinting, not only are we unbeatable, we are a joy to behold. Even when we do not win, we lose in style. Sometimes it's not whether you win or lose but how you run for your life.

Economics

You are the quickest in the village: a higher school wants you on its team. This is a ticket to college; the recruiters visit, the conditions are met – you run for your life. You learn from and you survive - the injuries, the offers. The opportunities are few, your family is poor; this may be your best chance to own something. You run for your life – you run for your living!

Administration and Volunteerism

You ran and you love running; in fact, you know the "runnings". You have trained, now you coach. Soon, to become part of the engine of running, you plan, you organize, you mentor. You volunteer because you love running; you live for running. You run – running for your *life*!

Belief

There are some things that come true when repeated. From birth we hear (1) all things are possible – *only believe*; (2) belief kills and belief cures. Every Jamaican believes this. Our belief is highlighted not only at Christmas but also during the annual hurricane season. During the week we run to school; on Sunday we run to church. This is easily translated into a strong belief in self. That is why we run like *lightning* whenever we run for our lives.

CHAPTER 12

The Challenge of Teaching Physical Education in Jamaica

VILMA CHARLTON

Teaching any subject in Jamaican schools is a challenge, but teaching children physical education is probably the most challenging of all, especially at the primary level. But despite the obstacles that confront all teachers, there is also the satisfaction to be gleaned from a job well done and the achievement of objectives. One main obstacle experienced by physical education teachers is the widespread concept of physical education as expendable, resulting in its Cinderella treatment and lack of the recognition accorded other subjects. If there is to be a special programme or an emergency meeting on any school day, the physical education period will be the one used, since school administrators tend to believe that this is the one class where children will not be losing out on any valuable information.

The scope of the work done in physical education is tremendous. In a single day, a high school physical edu-cation teacher may work with as many as seven classes of children. Their ages range from ten to sixteen years; their physical abilities from poor to excellent; their needs and interests from high interest in sports and physical fitness to the lack of interest manifested by those who have already decided that physical activity is not for them.

Origin and Meaning of Physical Education

Physical education, in some form or other, is as old as the human race. Primitive societies employed it mainly for survival and group unity. But they also utilized it for recreational purposes. There has been much contro-versy as to what to call this aspect of education and as to what it should comprise. The ancient Greeks called it "gymnastics", as did the Germans and other Euro-peans in the nineteenth century. The term "physical training" was used by the military, and "physical culture" was the term used in the latter part of the nineteenth century.

The term "physical education" developed as a protest against the formal activities of gymnastics with its formal method of teaching and is a more descriptive term mirroring its current objectives. Physical education enables individuals to express themselves through creative forms of activity and participation and promotes joy as well as reflective thinking and self-discipline. It includes vigorous activities, sports and games for the development of strength, skill and endurance; rhythmical activities and dance for the development of poise, skilful movement, social grace and artistic expression.

Physical education was first introduced in the army sometime after the Great War of 1918 and was then known as drill. It consisted of isolated and regimental-type exercises performed to precision in straight lines, under the direction of an instructor. The exercises were performed rhythmically, as in the army, and great care was taken to synchronize the movements. Physical education, introduced into Jamaica in the early twentieth century, received a boost in 1944, when two supervisors of physical training, I.G.P. Hughs and a Miss Bach from Great Britain, were provided under the Colonial Development and Welfare Act for the improvement and modernization of physical training throughout the schools of Jamaica.

The then-director of education, B.H. Easter, thereupon organized a conference of heads of training colleges to draw up a programme for physical training in the teacher training colleges. Subsequently, in-service training courses in physical training were conducted at various centres throughout the island; syllabuses for infant, lower, middle and upper divisions, as they were then called, were compiled and distributed to the infant and elementary schools for the guidance of teachers. These syllabuses were based on the historic 1933 syllabus of physical training in England. At the expiration of the contracts of Hughs and Bach, two supervisors, a male, Alvin Harper, and a female, Ivy Baxter, were appointed to continue the programme in Jamaica. The curriculum then consisted of physical exercises, cricket, netball, major games, athletics, and some folk and country dancing.

By the early 1950s, in-service teachers were being awarded scholarships annually to pursue one-year supplementary courses in physical education under the British Commonwealth Scholarship Scheme. One such teacher, Cynthia Walters, joined the Ministry of Education as education officer for physical education in 1956. Since then, the scope for physical education has been widened and now embraces a comprehensive range of physical activities including movement education; educational gymnastics; games – major and minor; athletics – track and field; dance – modern educational and folk, among others; aquatics – swimming and lifesaving; and camping and hiking.

By the early 1970s, the Physical Education Department became a part of the Cultural Arts Section in the ministry, with three officers, including a Jamaican dance specialist, Sheila Barnett. Subsequently, she was seconded to the Cultural Training Centre (now the Edna Manley College for the Visual and Performing Arts) as director of the School of Dance, where she trained teachers as specialists in this field. During the 1980s, Paul Cullingford, an expatriate from England, and Vilma Charlton, a Jamaican, were the two officers responsible for the physical education programme. It is therefore disturbing to note that in 1998 there was only one officer, Sonia Burke, to serve the whole island. In the year 2010 with the varied programmes in our schools and our successes in sport generally, there is still only one education officer, Dr Joyce Graham-Royal.

The Objectives of Physical Education

Many students frequently raise questions such as the following: How will physical education help me? What am I supposed to get out of physical education? Why can't I use the time for physical education to better advantage in studying the more important subjects? Too often no attempt is made to answer these serious queries. Consequently, many students often flounder aimlessly in their physical education classes. They are never introduced to the educational reasons for physical education programmes and what they are supposed to accomplish. What is far worse, they often receive an erroneous or one-sided view of physical education.

An educational programme of physical education can contribute to all the aspects and phases of individual development, although it contributes much more to certain aspects than to others. Its objectives can be considered under five categories: physical fitness, motor skills, knowledge, social objectives and aesthetic objectives.

Physical Fitness

As its name implies, physical education's chief contribution to an individual's education is in the area of the physical. The most important of its objectives is the attainment of physical fitness, which must not, however, be confused with the mere avoidance of illness. There should also be a sparkle and buoyancy to living. Physical fitness means the ability to carry one's workload without staggering, to participate in forms of recreation with ease and enjoyment, and to have a reservoir of endurance to meet the emergencies of life. In any occupation or profession, many crises often demand extra effort, and there should be adequate physical strength to meet them.

Properly directed, physical activity helps maintain the body in good health. While exercise cannot prevent or cure disease, it is a well-known medical fact that a person in run-down physical condition is more susceptible to illness and recovers more slowly. Exercise, used wisely, helps keep the body from getting into this state of lowered resistance. It builds up the muscles and vital organs of the body so that they are capable of taking more strain and consequently are kept at a higher level of efficiency. Health, therefore, is more than freedom from physical disease.

Health also includes mental health, to which physical education can contribute. Participation in a sport or game can take one's thoughts away from oneself. Life's problems can often be forgotten during a game, and the participant emerges tired in body but refreshed in spirit. It is difficult to measure the effectiveness of exercise in preventing mental illness, yet most authorities agree that exercise can be helpful. It is also true that sport and games, and even dancing, are widely used in treating certain types of mental illness. Bellevue Hospital for the mentally ill, in Kingston, Jamaica's capital, used to include dance sessions in its programme.

Motor Skills

To enjoy any occupation or activity, a person must achieve a certain amount of proficiency in it. Thus, one primary objective of physical education is learning the skills necessary to participate in sport. In addition, students in physical education classes should strive to acquire certain safety skills, vitally important in modern society. The skills of life-saving, protecting the body in falling, peripheral vision, coordination of mind with body and many others can be developed to varying degrees through the physical education programme.

Knowledge

At first glance, it may seem that there is little mental content in physical education. The fact is quite to the contrary, however, for we must learn the rules before we can learn to play a game. Once we know the rules and have achieved a certain proficiency in the activity, we often become interested in learning the strategy of the game. This mastery of strategy greatly facilitates the making of split-second decisions – excellent preparation for the actualities of life.

Social Objectives

Recent emphasis in education has been on improving the ability of students to get along. This culminated in 1994 in the formation of PALS (Peace and Love in Schools), an organization which helps children learn to resolve conflicts peacefully. In this age of social conflict, this objective is an important one. In sport, individuals must learn to exhibit the same qualities that are necessary for a successful and happy life in a democratic society. They must acquire attitudes and habits of loyalty, cooperation, initiative, self-control and courtesy. They learn to adapt themselves to constantly changing conditions of the game, just as they must in the game of life.

Aesthetic Objectives

In the field of physical education, the aesthetic objectives may be confined to three general areas: (1) appre-

ciation of exercise and its aesthetic effect on the body, (2) appreciation of sports and (3) appreciation of the wise use of leisure. Everybody admires a person who walks with grace and ease, a person who moves effortlessly, who maintains a youthful figure. All these qualities are available to all of us to a certain degree through regular and systematic participation in sports and physical games. Regular exercise can contribute to a healthy lifestyle.

Physical Education in Jamaica

The aim of the physical education programmes of the Ministry of Education in Jamaica is to provide and implement a programme designed to meet the developmental needs of the children of Jamaica. These needs are as follows:

1. Organic needs such as developing and maintaining strength and endurance.
2. Neuromuscular needs such as developing skills, grace in posture and efficiency of movement.
3. Personal and social needs such as developing self-confidence, leadership and intelligent followership, cooperation and emotional control.
4. Intellectual needs such as understanding the benefits of physical education, and knowing and understanding the rules and etiquette of each sport.
5. Emotional response needs such as experiencing the joy or pleasure of physical activity, meeting the challenge of hard work, experiencing satisfaction from personal efforts, experiencing new ideas and feeling adequate in social situations.

The minister of education maintains that physical education is the practical laboratory where students can practise many of the health concepts learned from day to day, and of course, daily physical activity is a most important basic health need.

The areas of emphasis are as follows:

1. Improving physical environments, such as the playfield, changing rooms if there are any, showers, toilets, activity rooms or gyms.
2. Adjusting classes to meet health needs, such as grouping according to developmental needs, wherever possible.
3. Adjusting rooms to meet health needs, such as physical space, light and ventilation.
4. Emphasizing personal appearance, cleanliness and grooming.
5. Emphasizing those attitudes and behavioural patterns that promote the positive qualities needed to live a good life.
6. Helping children understand their bodies – structure, function and proper care.
7. Teaching disease prevention and the correction of physical defects.
8. Discussing the relationship of certain health practices to prevention and control of disease, including the common cold, for example, the benefits of balanced diets, regular health check-ups, adequate sleep and rest, exercise and immunization.

Some of these areas still need attention, and the physical education unit of the Ministry of Education is continuing to address them.

Organization of Physical Education in Schools and Institutions

Infant and Basic Schools: Ages 4 to 5

Formal physical education lessons are not given at the infant level. A daily period of movement activity of 15 to 20 minutes is recommended for each child. Classes are coeducational and are led by the class teacher. The aim is to provide integrated curriculum experiences at this level and as far as the lower primary level.

Primary Schools: Grades 1 to 6

Classes are still coeducational at this level; physical education is taught by the classroom teacher, for two or three periods of 25 to 35 minutes weekly. In the upper grades (3 to 6), basic skills are introduced to form the foundations for sport and games such as netball, volleyball, cricket and football.

All-Age Schools: Grades 1 to 9

The programme for grades 1 to 6 in all-age schools is the same as for primary schools. In grades 7 to 9, the upper grades, classes are given separately for girls and boys, the girls being taught usually, though not always, by female teachers, the boys by male teachers. Due to the lack of facilities and trained teachers, this goal has not been reached in some schools.

Secondary Schools: Grades 7 to 11

In the secondary school, physical education classes are taught by specialist teachers and emphasize sports and games as well as fitness exercise for boys in particular.

Unfortunately, some of these schools organize special training programmes for the gifted, often at the expense of those with average ability. Dance and creative and expressive movements are taught mainly to girls. However, a few boys turn out to be potential dancers. A few secondary schools provide swimming instruction for selected pupils. Privately run swim clubs are also making their contribution by teaching and coaching youngsters of all ages. For those who show potential, development meets are organized.

Teachers' Colleges

Three of the eight teachers' colleges in Jamaica offer specialist training in physical education for student teachers in the secondary programme, and two of the colleges have fully equipped gymnasia. The others offer courses suitable for student teachers in the primary programme.

G.C. Foster College

The G.C. Foster College of Physical Education and Sport was established in September 1980 at Angels, St Catherine, Jamaica. This coeducational institution is the only one of its kind in the English-speaking Caribbean, and the original buildings and equipment were gifts of the Cuban government to the people of Jamaica. The college's main objective is to train specialist teachers of physical education. The training spans three academic years, or six semesters, and the final award is a diploma giving qualified-teacher status to students who successfully complete the programme. G.C. Foster College also offers a two-year certificate programme in physical education and sport for coaches.

In 1995, Jamaica attained another first in the field of sport, when G.C. Foster College became the first institution in the English-speaking Caribbean to offer a degree in physical education. The Bachelor of Physical Education (BPE) degree is accredited by the University Council of Jamaica. G.C. Foster College maintains close links with other tertiary institutions.

In 2008, the G.C. Foster College, in association with the University of Technology, Jamaica (UTech), began offering for the first time in Jamaica, a Master of Science degree in sports administration.

In-service Teacher Education Courses

Between 1973 and 1989, the Ministry of Education ran some intensive programmes of in-service training for teachers. The programme offered training courses for pre-trained teachers as well as refresher courses for qualified teachers to upgrade their skills both in physical activity and in actual teaching. These courses ranged from two- to three-day workshops to two- to three-week residential summer courses.

Curriculum Development

The Curriculum Development Unit of the Ministry of Education has revised the curriculum for all grades in the school system, writing curriculum guides, selecting reference books and recommending support materials. An effort is being made to integrate subject areas. Several projects have stimulated further development.

Since 1991 the Reform of Secondary Education (ROSE) project has triggered the reform of the curriculum at this level and has challenged teachers to become more creative and resourceful in their teaching. The

Primary Education Improvement Programme (PEIP) has attempted to bring a new philosophy to the teaching at this level. For example, themes taught in physical education are to be followed up by teachers in the classroom, and vice versa. Physical education specialists are to work with classroom teachers to organize lessons designed to follow up the physical education lesson taught the day before. The question is, Will the classroom teachers actually follow them? More important, though, physical education lessons themselves are to reflect and support the themes identified in the curriculum. In 2004 the Primary Education Support Project (PESP) was introduced as revision of the Joint Board of Teacher Education Primary Physical Education Programme.

The Ministry of Education realized in 2006 that not all teachers-in-training were exposed to all the aesthetic areas. It has now become mandatory that all student teachers receive some formal training in physical education, visual arts, and music and drama, though not in depth.

Scholarships

From time to time, one-year and three-year scholarships are awarded to practising teachers to upgrade their knowledge and skills and qualify themselves at institutions such as Leeds University, Bedford College, East Sussex College, and Nedlands College, Australia. These have now become infrequent. However, the Cuban government is about to open up new avenues for student teachers and coaches to pursue programmes or upgrade their training.

Competitions

Competitions are organized by schools and colleges on intramural, zone, parish and all-island levels. Activities include track and field, netball, volleyball, football, cricket and swimming. These competitions are now heavily sponsored by the private sector. Jamaica may be the only country that offers regular formal competitions for boys and girls at the high-school level, contributing to the richness of our results in world-class events. In 2010 Jamaica will celebrate one hundred years of the running of Boys' Championships. Although the girls' have merged with the boys' high schools, they began their all-island competitions in the early 1950s. The early childhood schools and the primary schools all have similar championships.

Difficulties

Physical education teachers in the secondary schools have heavy workloads. They have full timetables and have to deal with adolescents in all their variety of characteristics and dispositions. In addition, many of these teachers have programmes after school, and a few swim coaches have classes or training before school, in the mornings.

Now that physical education is being offered as a CXC subject, since 2005, schools have difficulty getting slots on their timetable to teach the relevant courses. A number of teachers therefore must teach after school to get through the syllabus.

The primary school teacher may have a lighter programme, as very often each grade is timetabled for only one period a week. But this teacher may be faced with other obstacles, having perhaps to deal with a greater class size in which many of the children are uncoordinated. This teacher often does not have enough equipment for use in any one class.

Few teachers can complete their days under anything close to ideal circumstances. The playfields are usually dusty or stony, or even nonexistent, so physical education may be taught in halls, lobbies, classrooms and, for others, on stages inside or outside a hall. Some classroom teachers insist on keeping the students beyond their assigned class time when they realize that physical education is the class following. Others use the time allotted for physical education as a "catch-up" for remedial work in mathematics and reading. The feeling persists that physical education is not important. Adult persons remembering the physical education classes of their school days think they still feature only games such as dodge-ball, bull-in-the-pen and scrimmage. This is particularly hard on those children who truly enjoy physical education. Adults often do not understand how things have changed since they were in school.

Benefits

Clearly, the chief benefit of teaching is not the salary. The really dedicated physical education teachers work after school with school clubs and teams at no extra cost to the education system. Their summers are often spent attending teaching or coaching seminars locally or internationally, and are not, as perceived, two months of rest and recuperation.

One of the most obvious benefits for the physical education teacher is simply the joy of being with children – the laughs, the hugs, the "thank you Miss/Sir for listening to my problem," the trust in their Miss or Sir,

the break from the classroom routine, the smiles when a new skill is tried and mastered, and the opportunity to introduce children to lifetime values, skills, health and leisure time activities. These small rewards occur frequently and are sometimes the most meaningful. As long as teachers remain sensitive to the children, there are few jobs that they can find as gratifying.

Another benefit that occurs less frequently is the satisfaction of seeing children grow and develop. It is humbling for a teacher who has remained at the same school for five or six years to observe his or her classes and school teams, and realize that much of what these children know or do not know is a direct result of the teacher's physical education programme.

The Need for Planning

Only a few teachers would question the importance of planning for effective physical education classes. The question, however, is how much planning is necessary. At the beginning of their careers, teachers need to spend more time planning than they do once they have gained experience. This is no different from taking a trip for the first time. Here one has to study maps and landmarks to know exactly where to go. After the trip has been made several times, however, far less time needs to be spent reviewing maps.

The amount of planning necessary is related to the type of programme a teacher decides to provide for children. Teachers who "throw out the ball" and send children to play while they sit in the staff room or run an errand will probably spend no more than ten minutes a week thinking about what they will teach.

On the other hand, teachers who try to put a good programme together spend considerable time creating and organizing lessons that fulfil the needs of their pupils. They sometimes invite resource persons to add even more excitement to the programme.

Actual Class Time

One major reason why planning is crucial is that minimum time is given to physical education in schools. A primary grade which receives thirty minutes for a physical education class each week will never have enough time to cover and learn all the prescribed skills. Within these thirty-minute classes at the primary level, time is spent before and after class changing into and out of the school uniforms, reducing the length of the period by several minutes. This subject has numerous areas, and each area covers many technical skills which ought to be fairly well mastered if playing or participating in sport is to be enjoyed.

The secondary grades may have two to three periods of physical education a week, each forty-five minutes long; sometimes there is a double period of ninety minutes. This is still not enough time, given the variety of activities and the sport and games played in competitions. One difference at this level, though, is that the secondary schools may have more than one physical education specialist teacher, while the primary schools normally use the classroom teacher or one who has had some training in their college programme – neither of whom is likely to be specialist in physical education.

In 1996, the National Sports Council proposed that specialist physical education graduates should be allowed to teach at the primary level. Should this proposal, taken to Cabinet and passed, be put into effect and become operational, we could begin to see a difference in the organization and stature of physical education at the primary level. According to the document "National Sports Policy for Jamaica", the Ministry of Education is expected to ensure that the curricula of all schools include physical education and that adequate time is provided for the practice of sport. Schools with an enrolment of six hundred and over are to have a full-time qualified physical education teacher, and smaller schools are to be organized in groups or clusters for similar assistance. In the last few years many schools have begun the process of hiring a full-time teacher at the primary level.

Teaching Environment

Apart from the limited amount of time, many other factors influence the physical education programme. Class size, equipment and facilities all determine what can be taught successfully. The climate, too, is a factor which can affect physical education lessons, as it may be too hot or too rainy. On rainy days, classes are held inside tiny classrooms surrounded by desks and chairs or in a hall. Teachers are encouraged to prepare rainy day activities. The variety and quality of physical education equipment available on the market have improved considerably, but their effective use requires careful planning.

Staff Development

Teachers often have to teach aspects of the programme with which they are unfamiliar. They therefore need to spend much more time in planning and developing the expertise to teach these activities effectively. Some teachers enrich their backgrounds through reading materials. Others attend conferences, workshops or seminars. Some ask other teachers for practical help or they may invite guest lecturers. Teachers also attend workshops held by the governing sporting bodies.

Larry Horine (1991) placed great emphasis on staff development. In his view, "If everything is done to employ the best staff, the most effective way of improving performance is through staff development." For Horine, "staff development includes individual and group efforts; it encompasses any planned or unplanned activity that results in improved performance. This might mean eliminating personal problems or learning a technical skill such as a new teaching method."

Some of our teachers now receive journals and magazines from overseas associations such as those from Canada and the United States. Whereas the secondary teachers may specialize in certain areas of physical education, the primary school physical education teachers are expected to be an expert in virtually every aspect of physical education. This means that they often need to find ways to learn about new activities or activities that were neglected in our teacher preparation programme, so that they can offer children a complete and well-rounded programme. For them, then, staff development becomes even more essential.

The Teacher Can Make the Difference

Physical education teachers are really no different from teachers of any other subject. They want their students to learn. They also want them to enjoy their classes. Some physical education teachers emphasize the learning of motor skills and the playing of games. Others emphasize the development of physical fitness and competition in each sport. Some place their major emphasis on the development of positive student attitudes towards themselves and towards the subject of physical education. Of course, many teachers would

use a combination of these programmes. It is quite easy to list goals for a programme but it can be difficult to accomplish these goals, especially when classes are large and the number of class periods is limited to one, two or three days a week.

A successful programme should encourage children to learn and to develop positive attitudes towards the subject. It should also help teachers to gain satisfaction from their jobs. Most important, physical education programmes can be successful only if the programmes are in line with the overall goals and focus of the school.

Obstacles

The physical education programme in Jamaican schools has been hampered by the following major obstacles:

1. Although the private sector and the Ministry of Education provide for further development of teachers in service, the number of ministry-based personnel to supervise the work in the schools is inadequate.
2. Although there has been some improvement, there is a shortage of qualified physical education teachers in the schools.
3. Playfields are hot, dusty, stony or nonexistent.
4. Physical education is not treated as a compulsory subject in the schools.
5. The physical education grant and the actual equipment are inadequate. Currently, the infant, primary and all-age schools receive basic equipment, while the secondary schools receive an allocation of approximately $2 per capita.
6. The attrition rate of physical education teachers is high. This is largely due to the inadequacy of the provision for physical education.

The following suggestions are offered to remove the obstacles:

1. That physical education be made compulsory in all schools.
2. That all schools be built with a covered area for physical education. It is unbearable to teach and learn for long hours in the tropical sun.
3. That schools aim at building as many permanent facilities as possible and building up their supplies of equipment. Such projects could be financed by the ministry through grants, fund-raising and private sector assistance.
4. That itinerant teachers having special expertise in some area of physical education such as movement education, dance or volleyball be appointed to work in groups of schools.
5. That the government plan to build more permanent facilities such as stadia placed in and around the counties – Surrey, Middlesex and Cornwall. Outside of Kingston and St Catherine there is one stadium in Cambridge, Montego Bay, and another – though it has no track, only a cricket pitch – is in Greenfield, Trelawny. Congratulations to the University of the West Indies, Mona, and, in particular, Olympian Grace Jackson and coach Glen Mills, who, along with Usain Bolt and PUMA, received a track (a gift to Bolt) from Regupol. This was the same type of track on which Usain Bolt ran his three world records at the Beijing Olympic Games in China.

These proposals could remove many of the obstacles teachers encounter in implementing the physical education programme in Jamaican schools. If these obstacles are dealt with, our successes in sport generally would be resounding.

Acknowledgements

The original version of this chapter was published in the *Institute of Education Annual: The Challenge of Teaching Physical Education,* vol. 1, ed. Ruby King (Kingston: Institute of Education, University of the West Indies, 1998), 128–40.

References

Government of Jamaica. 1979. Report from the International Conference on Physical Education and Sports. Government of Jamaica and UNESCO.

Graham, G. 1992. *Teaching children physical education.* Champaign, IL: Human Kinetics.

Horine, L. 1991. *Administration of physical education and sports programs.* Dubuque, IA: William C. Brown.

CHAPTER 13

The Role of Boys' and Girls' Championships in Jamaica's Track-and-Field Glory

INTERVIEW WITH BOBBY FRAY BY VILMA CHARLTON AND FRED GREEN

Sports historian Bobby Fray reminisces with Olympian Vilma Charlton and retired sports administrator Fred Green.

Bobby Fray: In our opening lines we would like to pay eternal credit to some of our founding fathers and mothers who came in various guises. These were, first of all, the early visionary headmasters and head-mistresses who exemplified the words of the Bible: "Without vision the people perish."

These sterling principals in the early and mid-twentieth century recognized that it was important to lay a sound academic framework, but they did not merely stop there. These early stalwarts took excruciating care to incorporate the words of the Latin maxim *mens sana in corpore sano* (translated: "a sound mind in a healthy body").

Further reduced to its simplest form, it could be said of these early educators that they thought all work and

no play would make Jack or Jill a dull boy or dull girl. This was done without sacrificing the fundamentals of academics for which school girls and school boys went to secondary schools, or what are known as high or technical schools.

Thus, it was that our very first female finalist in the 100 metres at our debut Olympic Games 1948, in London, England, Cynthia Thompson, was to become later in life a medical doctor, after attending one of Jamaica's prestigious educational institutions, St Hugh's High School.

In collaborative efforts in writing this chapter, Dr Cynthia Thompson has opined that she left St Hugh's in 1940, and she recalls that the first attempt at a competitive championship for girls did not come about until

1941, the year after her departure from high school.

Howsoever, if the cynics – and remember, there are always detractors – wish to point out that Dr Thompson did not cut (is this the expression?) her eye-teeth or eye-tooth in the rough and tumble of a Girls' Athletic Championship (Champs), the same can't be said on the boys' side. I am coming to Arthur Wint now.

There is incontrovertible evidence that Arthur Wint of Calabar High School and Excelsior High School, who became our first individual Olympic medallist in 1948, as well as our very first Olympic gold medallist that same year, not only competed at Boys' Championships but was eminently successful.

Arthur Wint was a gold medallist at Boys' Champs from the initial stage of competition, that is, at the under-fourteen stage, which is referred to as class 3.

As was the case with Dr Thompson, whom he preceded, Arthur Wint became a medical doctor and was later to become the founding president of the invaluable and seminal organization, the Sports Medicine Association of Jamaica.

Dr Arthur Wint not only competed very well in our first Olympics in London, England, but during his academic studies in that country, was invited to captain Great Britain's track and field teams in friendly internationals. History will also recall that Dr Arthur Wint, a personable and well-rounded individual, certainly at the level of the Central American and Caribbean Games (CAC), was one of the most versatile athletes to represent Jamaica, or any other country, for that matter.

In his later years, Dr Arthur Wint also distinguished himself as a diplomatic ambassador to Great Britain and served as senior medical officer for health (SMO) in his homeland. I am trying to put up a point for sports.

To make a sixteen-year leap forward in history, Una Morris, who was to become Dr Una Morris-Chong, not only competed at the 1964 Olympic Games in Tokyo, Japan, at the tender age of sixteen years but made a significant and telling contribution on and off the track. Una Morris excelled at the Tokyo Olympic Games, placing fourth in the 200 metres.

Una, at the time of her Olympic Games exploits, was a student of Jamaica's first technical high school, Kingston Technical High School, situated in the downtown sector of the capital city, Kingston. Una was produced locally in Jamaica by track and field coach Noel White.

Una Morris, as was earlier adverted to, attended a technical high school, but this did not prevent her from becoming a career medical doctor, a radiologist to boot.

On the subject of Jamaican lasses competing at the highest level of sports at tender ages, we fast-forward another sixteen years to the Moscow Olympic Games of 1980. It was in the USSR where the 1980 Olympic Games were staged that we had two other instances of the precocious nature of Jamaica's track and field. It was in that edition of the Olympic Games that Juliet Cuthbert of Morant Bay High School from the eastern parish of St Thomas emerged for what was to be a distinguished Olympic career.

Juliet participated in five Olympic Games – 1980, 1984, 1988, 1992 and 1996 – a feat exceeded only by the phenomenal Merlene Joyce Ottey, who figured in an unprecedented six Olympic Games for Jamaica – 1980 to 2000 – as well as a seventh Olympics for her adopted country of Slovenia, in the 2004 Olympic Games. Jamaica's sportswoman of the year for 1992, Juliet Cuthbert was also to make an erudite main address. Juliet was also excellently prepared at high school by educator Howard Jackson, who became principal of Morant Bay High School.

Sadly, Howard Jackson, who would have seen Juliet Cuthbert's fabulous exploits at the 1992 Olympic Games in Barcelona, Spain, where she was to garner two splendid silver medals in the 100 and 200 metres, was to die prematurely.

The then-president of the Jamaica Amateur Athletic Association (JAAA), Mr Neville Teddy McCook, had appointed Mr Jackson to be a part of Jamaica's coaching contingent at the 1993 edition of the World Championship in Stuttgart, Germany, but as events turned out, his untimely passing prevented him taking up the appointment.

Another sixteen-year-old entrant in the 1980 Olympic Games in Moscow was Cathy Rattray.

Vilma Charlton: She started at Excelsior and then finished in Washington, where her father was the Jamaican ambassador.

BF: Cathy competed in the 400 metres and the 4 × 100-metre relay and overall competed in four Olympic Games. Juliet Cuthbert finished high school in the United States and later attended the University of Texas. Cathy Rattray attended the University of Tennessee.

At the outset of this article we opined that Jamaica's profound success in track and field was due in part to the early acclaimed, path-finding leadership of the principals of both genders. One would be remiss not to mention that these educators whose primary duties were to micro-manage the academic affairs of their students would not have been able to achieve and attain the veritable successes that they did without a far-reaching institution known as the Inter-secondary Schools Sports Association (ISSA) and a creature and offshoot of that organization known as the ISSA secretary-general.

An outstanding example is Mr Harry H.N. "Chicken" Walker, who later became principal of the venerable Wolmer's Boys' School, founded in 1729. Another tremendous holder of the post of secretary-general of ISSA was Mr W. Fred Green. In his administrative endeavours in track and field, Mr Green has also been accorded awards from the International Amateur Athletic Federation, the IAAF. Mr W. Fred Green served as secretary-general of ISSA for an extended period.

Fred Green: Before you go on, talk about Champs Centenary.

BF: It is nothing short of being absolutely remarkable that, in 2010, ISSA will celebrate the centenary of Boys' Athletic Championships. How many nations can boast of one hundred years of frenetic track and field activity? If this is not a true indicator of insightful administrative minds, of first rate leadership, then I do not know what is.

We must not forget that we have had qualitative athletes and personnel from the inception. One case springs readily to mind: Norman Washington Manley, born 4 July 1893, who was an early *victor ludorum*. That is, champion boy with unparalleled feat of versatility. And, for example, the 100 yards in which Manley ran 10 seconds flat would have placed him in the finals of the 1912 Olympic Games. A debilitating viral illness took away his snappiness and sharpness as a top-flight athlete. The outbreak of the First World War (1914 to 1919) further eroded his track and field excellence at the top, but did not prevent N.W. Manley from earning a military medal for distinguished service in the war.

Nothing also prevented meritorious service as a Jamaican Rhodes scholar at Oxford University, England, and tireless advocacy as a lawyer and outstanding public servant, especially as chief minister and premier of

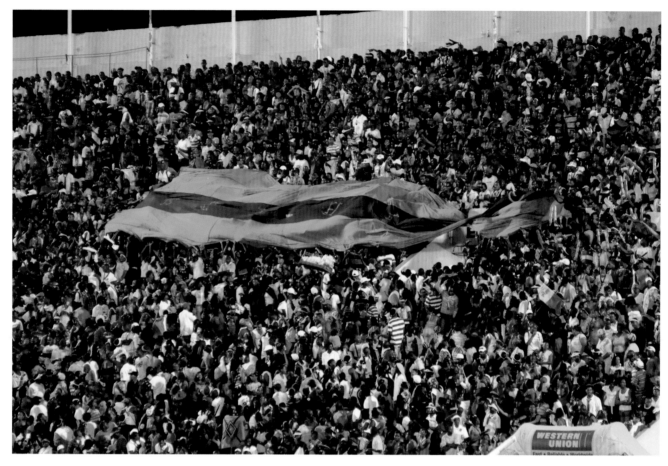

PLATE 13.1 The competitive spirit is fanned at Boys' Championships by the intense rivalry between the top-performing schools and the tremendous support they enjoy at each staging of the championships. Crowd pictured in 2009 supporting Calabar (green). (*Jamaica Observer* photograph.)

Jamaica, 1955 to 1962, and as a key member of the fledgling and ill-fated West Indies Federation, 1958 to 1961. So, in other words, it must be remembered that it was Mr Manley who gave the go-ahead as premier for the construction of the National Stadium, which was built in 1962. Another key area of contribution to Jamaican life by N.W. Manley was as president of the Jamaica Amateur Athletic Association and as president

of the Jamaica Boxing Board of Control. The observation has to be made that the work of the Inter-secondary Schools Sports Association in later years was emboldened by the formation the Jamaica Amateur Athletic Association, as a guiding parental light in athletics. The JAAA has since been served by a succession of quite outstanding presidents, executives who have led to Jamaica's participation at the senior level in the

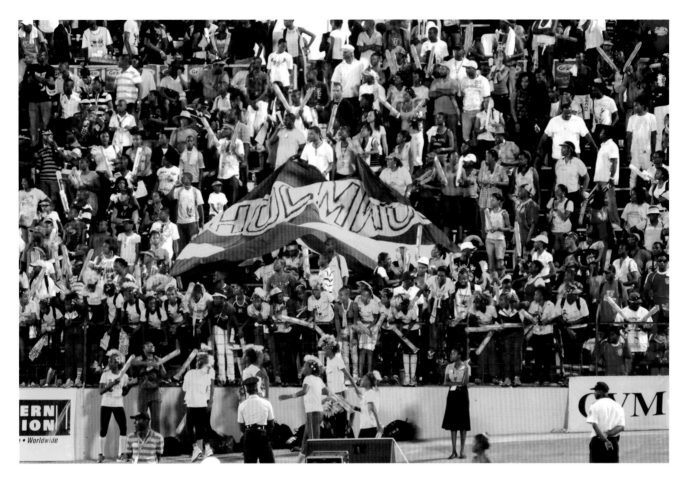

PLATE 13.2 Fans and students from Holmwood Technical High School raising the school's flag. Holmwood girls, in recent times, have being a dominant force at the annual Boys' and Girls' Championships. (*Jamaica Observer* photograph.)

Olympic Games, the World Championships, World Indoors, athletic World Cup and University Games, as well as involvement in the Commonwealth Games, the Pan American Games and the Central American and Caribbean Games.

At the junior level there has been involvement of Jamaica's athletes at the World Junior Championships, the World Youth Championships, the Junior Pan American Athletic Championships (which started in 1980), the Junior Central American and Caribbean, CAC American Championships and the Junior Carifta Games, which had its inaugural outing in Bridgetown, Barbados, in 1972. We forget at our peril the vital roles played by members and the president of Jamaica's premier sporting body, the Jamaica Olympic Association (JOA).

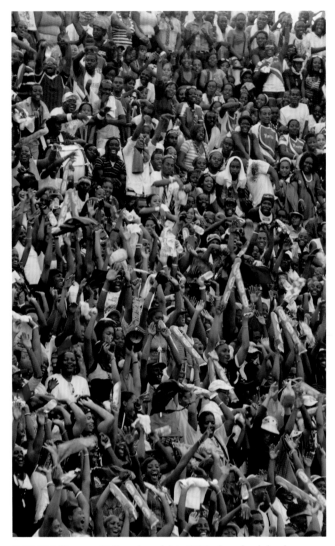

PLATE 13.3 Kingston College (purple) in 2009, the school that has enjoyed the most victories through the hundred years of competition. (*Jamaica Observer* photograph.)

Some of the outstanding presidents of the JOA include His Excellency Mr Tony Bridge, who graduated to being a member of the International Olympic Committee (IOC), as well as Sir Herbert MacDonald, who was head of the organizing committee when Jamaica

hosted the ninth CAC Games at the new National Stadium in 1962, days after the attainment of political independence on 6 August. Sir Herbert MacDonald was also chairman of the organizing committee when Jamaica had the national honour of housing the eighth Commonwealth Games in Kingston in 1966.

FG: At that time it was called the British Empire and Commonwealth Games.

BF: We as a little nation weren't even supposed to be there. Our worthies who have served the JOA have been Mr Keith Shervington and the incumbent head of the JOA since 1977, Mr Mike Fennel, who is also the long-standing president of the Commonwealth Games Federation.

VC: Yes, we are proud of him.

BF: Vinton Beckett came fourth in the high jump in 1948, and then I want to make the point that women were treated as the poor relation in athletics, and that, more than anything, was why it took thirty-two years to move from fourth place for women to the first of medals for women, one generation later, which was Merlene Joyce Ottey, getting a bronze in the 200 metres in Moscow in 1980.

VC: Was that because we didn't have strong support for Girls' Champs then as against the Boys'?

BF: That's the point I want to make. That it was the Girls' Champs which was started on or about 1941, but was discontinued after a certain period and not picked up until 1957, when it was St Hilda's who won the new version of the Girls' Championships. Included as outstanding members of that 1962 Girls' Championships were athletes such as Vilma Charlton, OD, who won both 100 and the 200 metres, was named *victrix ludo-*

rum and went on to attend three Olympic Games in 1964, 1968 and 1972. Miss Charlton was also a member of Jamaica's gold medal team which won the 4 × 100 metres at the 1962 and 1966 CAC Games.

VC: Talk about the impact of Boys' Champs on all our successes. Let's take the era of Herb McKenley and Arthur Wint. Did Champs have anything to do with their successes?

BF: As I said before, Arthur Wint went to Calabar and Excelsior High Schools. Herb McKenley ran for Calabar High School and competed in very competitive races with Leroy "Coco" Brown of Wolmer's Boys' school and Douglas Manley, son of the national hero and later to be a cabinet minister. Herbert McKenley was regarded by many as perhaps the greatest thing since sliced bread, but he had a very tough time crossing the line first at Boys' Champs, and *Sports Life* magazine recorded that the one time that Herb McKenley set a record at Champs, the track was found to have been just a wee bit short.

I am making the point now that whereas we have had Usain Bolt and we have had even Asafa Powell reaching a final of Boys' Championships, whereas we have had Wint, McKenley and Leslie Laing, who attended Dinthill Technical, we have also had a situation existing at Boys' Champs where Bertland Cameron, who was our first ever gold medallist at the World Championships in Helsinki in 1983, never crossed the line first at Boys' Champs. He was to come second in 1978 to Norman Hunter of Jamaica College. Bertland then went to the Commonwealth Games of 1978 and excelled. But in 1979, while competing at the Boys' Championships he equalled the record of 47.3 seconds in semi-final one, but Kingston College's Ian Stapleton was to run a record 46.6 seconds in the second semi-

final. In the final, while it was still touch-and-go between Cameron and Stapleton, Stapleton triumphed overall with a record of 46.2 seconds.

Both Cameron and Stapleton in that said year of 1979 went to the Pan American Games in San Juan, Puerto Rico, where Jamaica gained a silver medal in the 4 × 400-metre relay while both were still below age twenty years.

We have had situations such as Rupert Hoilett, who went to the 1964 Games in Tokyo as an alternate to the 4 × 400-metre team, which was one of four instances in which Jamaica placed fourth at the 1964 Tokyo Olympic Games. In other words, we came fourth in the women's 200 metres, George Kerr came fourth in the 800 metres. We came fourth in the 4 × 100 metres and fourth in the 4 × 400 metres. Injuries prevented Rupert Hoilett from progressing. He won the 400 metres three years in class 1 (1963, 1964 and 1965), setting a then-record in 1965 of 47.9 seconds. Injuries were to curtail his career.

VC: Speak about the outstanding athletes at Boys' Champs.

BF: We are coming to the late Lennox Miller now. Dr Lennox "Billy" Miller, a dentist, also won in, for three years, the 100 and 200 metres at Boys' Championships after he had been upset in the 100 metres in his last year in class 2. Both Miller and Hoilett were members of the Kingston College (KC) inaugural team which won gold as the first Jamaican team to go to the Penn Relays, where the Kingston College aggregation of coaches, such as Donovan Davis and Howard Avis were joined in an advisory capacity by Calabar's late great Herb McKenley, because KC asked Mr McKenley to accompany them.

I want to make the point that Lennox Miller, who

was a true Champs product, was our silver medallist in the 100 metres at the 1968 Olympic Games in Mexico City and a bronze medallist at the 1972 Olympic Games in Munich, Germany, at a time when he was concentrating on his dental studies.

Then another outstanding product of the Boys' Championships is Donald Quarrie, who competed and got better as he went on from classes 3 to 2 to 1. Donald Quarrie was also at those times running below 21 seconds for the 220 yards at Boys' Championships, which was an outstanding achievement, and it was in 1969 that he defeated Errol Stewart in a very competitive 100 yards at Boys' Championships, which is important because within one year they were to excel at the 1970 Commonwealth Games. In that 1970 Commonwealth Games Quarrie won the 100-metre gold and the 200-metre gold, and both he and Stewart were on the 4 × 100 metres gold medal team, which included Lennox Miller, the one 100-metre silver medallist, and Carl Lawson.

VC: This was about a decade after Dennis Johnson!

BF: In other words, Dennis Johnson of Calabar High School as long ago as 1958 set the then-championship records of 9.8 seconds and 21.8 seconds in the 100 yards and 220 yards at the Boys' Championships. In 1961 he equalled the 100 yards record of 9.3 seconds which he did on four occasions during the year 1961.

Raymond Stewart, who reached three consecutive Olympic Games (100-metre finals in 1984, 1988 and 1992), also competed very well at Boys' Championships. He was the 1983 and 1984 Boys' Champs 100 metres gold medallist, and, in fact, won his semi-final at the 1984 Olympic Games in Los Angeles, California, while he was still a student. In that same year that he

competed for Camperdown High School at the Boys' Championships.

The fourth member of Jamaica's silver-medal 4 × 100-metre team, the first male sprint team to get an Olympic medal, all went through the Champs programme. The team included Albert Lawrence of Vere Technical High School, Gregory Meghoo of St Jago High School, Donald Quarrie of Camperdown High School and Raymond Stewart also of Camperdown High School. Does that take us up to 1984?

VC: Speak also of the girls' contribution . . .

BF: Yes. We come back now to your sprint team of 1964. We reached the sprint final with you who competed for St Andrew High School, and Rosie Allwood, who competed for Titchfield High School, another of our venerable institutions. Rosie made the 1972 Olympic 200-metre final in Munich, Germany.

Another outstanding female prospect was Jacqueline Pusey who excelled at Girls' Champs in the 100 and the 200 metres for St Mary's High School. It had seemed, had injury not intervened, that perhaps she would have been a forerunner to the great Merlene Ottey.

Merlene Ottey won the sprint double at the 1979 Girls' Athletic Championships, although, ironically, she did not excel in the 1979 Carifta Games, which were held in Kingston, Jamaica, in that year, in the same year as the Pan American Games. In the senior Pan American Games in San Juan, Puerto Rico, she came third in the 200 metres, in a race won by the world's then-number-one sprinter, Evelyn Ashford of the United States of America. Merlene was to get a bronze medal and become the very first female athlete for the English-speaking Caribbean to get an Olympic medal.

It is ironic that all this acerbic or coarse talk of "Bronze Queen" may never have arisen had she not lost by one hundredth of a second to an athlete who set the then-World Junior Championship record. It is, however, interesting that Miss Ottey, maybe, has won monuments more lasting than bronze, that it is Merlene who survived and endured to last, as was previously adverted to, from 1980 to 2010.

Merlene represented Rusea's School, another of our old institutions, and also the institution which is perhaps Jamaica's most outstanding high school in producing Olympians, namely Vere Technical High School. Merlene has the record number of medals for any female athlete in the history of the Olympic Games. If her fourth place in the 100 metres at age forty years in the 2000 Sydney Olympic Games is upgraded to a bronze, it would mean that Ambassador Ottey would have nine Olympic medals. That would be three silver medals and six bronze medals.

Merlene Joyce Ottey also has fourteen medals from the World Championships, the most medals for any female athlete at the Championships. This is a special honour, as, when she started for the first three editions of those World Championships, they, like the Olympic Games, were held over a quadrennial, that is, a four-year period. So, for example, she ran in 1983, 1987 and 1991, but it was not until Stuttgart, Germany, in 1993, that the World Championships were reduced to twice-yearly events. Still, Ambassador Ottey has emerged with three gold medals. She has two individual gold medals in the 200 metres, one in Stuttgart, Germany, in 1993, and a repeat performance in Sweden in 1995. She took the baton in third position in the 1991 World Championships in Tokyo, Japan, and guided Jamaica to a then national record of 41.94 seconds and won gold in the 4 × 100-metre relay. So that would be three gold medals. In May 2010, Merlene turned fifty years old and is still competing.

VC: We already spoke about Juliet Cuthbert. What of the other women?

BF: Audrey Reid and Andrea Bruce, who is now a dental surgeon, were Olympic finalists in the high jump in 1968 and 1972. Since then, only Karen Beautle has gone to the world level and actually medalled. In 2006 Beautle won the bronze medal. Grace Jackson, who competed for Queen's School in 1978, but interestingly was an all-round athlete, competing in events such as the hurdles and the high jump, was to become the region's first female Olympic silver medallist. She did 21.72 seconds for the 200 metres to get the silver medal behind Florence Griffith-Joyner of the United States who set the world record of 21.34 seconds.

In 1992 Jamaica had three female entrants in the Olympic Games finals in Barcelona, Spain. Juliet Cuthbert who got a silver medal, Merlene Ottey who got a bronze medal and Grace Jackson who was a finalist. It is interesting to note that, once again, if Jamaica gets a medal out of Marion Jones's disqualification in the 2000 Olympics, then Jamaica would have an unbroken record since 1980 of winning a medal for the 200 metres at every Olympic Games – in other words, from 1980 to 2008. An unprecedented twenty-eight years.

It was in 1980 that Merlene got the bronze medal; in 1984 Merlene again got the bronze medal; in 1988 Grace Jackson got the silver medal. Merlene was fourth with a bandaged leg. In 1992, Juliet Cuthbert got the silver medal, and we previously mentioned what happened with the three Jamaican finalists. In 1996, Merlene got the silver medal in Atlanta. In 2000, Beverly McDonald, formerly of Vere Technical High School and one of our most prolific medal winners at the junior level, and also a member of the World Championship gold medal team of 1991, came fourth. So if Beverly's upgraded to a bronze, Jamaica would have a bronze in the 200 metres in 2000 due to Marion Jones's disqualification.

In 2004, Veronica Campbell, as she then was, became our first gold medallist in the 200 metres in the Olympic Games, with Aleen Bailey placing fourth. In 2008 Veronica Campbell-Brown, as she was to become, retained her title, becoming the second woman in history to repeat in the 200 metres. Kerron Stewart, another outstanding championship product from St Jago High School, got the bronze medal, with Sherone Simpson also reaching the final.

It is important to note that Veronica Campbell, who competed for and won the gold medal at the 2001 Girls' Championships in class 1, is also the only athlete to have won gold at the world youth level, that is, the competition for youngsters under eighteen years old. She has also won the 100 metres at the World Junior Championships, becoming the first woman to win the sprint double, the 100 and 200 metres at the World Junior Championships, then the first woman to follow up by winning the 100-metre gold at the World Senior Athletic Championships, which she did in Osaka, Japan, in 2007, which has given her a special lane at the World Championships in 2009, irrespective of what would have happened in that event at the Jamaica national trials of 2009.

So, it is also important that Sherone Simpson of Manchester High School, another Girls' Champs product, was a member of Jamaica's 4 × 100-metre team in the 2002 World Junior Championships in Kingston, Jamaica, which got gold. Sherone Simpson and Kerron Stewart, both Girls' Championships products, ended up with the silver medal, with the joint silver medal in the one 100 metres at the 2008 Olympic Games.

Needless to say, it was Wolmerian Shelly-Ann Fraser who had won at Girls' Champs in class 2, but never repeated the feat in class 1, who was to become the first ever English-speaking Caribbean woman to win the Olympic 100-metre gold, which she did in a fabulous time of 10.78 seconds. She later in 2009 did 10.73 seconds in the 100 metres at the World Championships, making her the fastest Jamaican woman.

VC: Can you refer to the boys in that period?

BF: Before I do, I should mention three girls who came out of it. At the lowest level there is Merlene Fraser, who came from Vere Technical High School at just seventeen years old, and was an alternate in the women's World Championships gold medal team of 1991.

Then there was Nikole Mitchell. St Jago's Melaine Walker was another outstanding product at the Girls' Athletic Championships, running with a broken arm in class 2 in 1999; Melaine beat the acclaimed Veronica Campbell not only in the 100 metres but in the 200 metres. In 2008, Melaine Walker won the gold in an Olympic record time of 52.64 seconds. This leads to another point that not one size fits all, and the first ever woman to win an Olympic gold medal for Jamaica or the English-speaking Caribbean was Deon Hemmings, now Deon Hemmings-McCatty, but interestingly, while she competed for York Castle High School and Vere Technical High School, she never won a gold medal at the Girls' Athletic Championships.

Nikole Mitchell first represented St Mary's High School under the coaching of Danny Hawthorne who was to bring Yohan Blake to early prominence. Yohan Blake set a national junior record in the men's 100 metres. Nikole Mitchell first went to St Mary's High School and then Wolmer's Girls School. Nikole was the 1992 World Junior Championship gold medallist in the

100 metres, having got the silver two years earlier in 1990 in Plovdiv, Bulgaria, at the age of fifteen years.

Gillian Russell, of Campion College, also competed at Girls' Championships, has the record number of gold medals at the World Junior Championships, winning the one 100-metre sprint hurdles in Bulgaria in 1990 and in Seoul, South Korea, in 1992. Both Gillian and Nikole started in the gold-medal-winning World Junior Championship 4 × 100-metre team in 1990. Nikole anchored the team and both have gold medals in the sprints at the World Junior Championships in 1990 and 1992. So therefore Gillian Russell has four World Junior Championship medals and Nikole Mitchell has three World Junior Championship gold medals and one silver medal.

While it took thirty-two years between Vinton Beckett getting fourth in the high jump at the Olympic Games in 1948 and Merlene getting a bronze in the 200 metres in 1980, we must not forget that Audrey Reid and Andrea Bruce, both of whom competed at Girls' Championships, reached the finals of the high jump at their respective Olympic Games.

Kathleen Russell was also a finalist in the 80-metre sprint hurdles, as it then was, in the 1948 Olympic Games in London, England. Carmen Phipps also distinguished herself on the 1948 Olympic team.

Let us talk about Usain and Asafa. It is no surprise that Usain Bolt, who holds the Boys' Championships class 1, 200-metre record of 20.25 seconds, and the 400-metre class 1 record of 45.35 seconds, also competed with distinction at the Boys' Championships, doing so for William Knibb Memorial High School in Trelawny.

Usain, like Veronica Campbell-Brown, was also a World Youth Champion and a World Junior Champion in the 200 metres. At the World Junior Championships

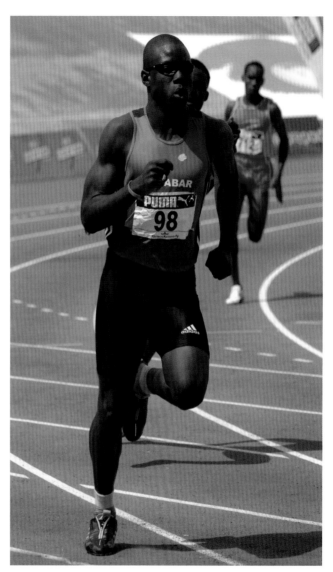

PLATE 13.4 Ramone McKenzie of Calabar was one of the top performers at Boys' Championships in 2009. He qualified for the Jamaican team and participated at the World Championships in Berlin. (*Gleaner* photograph.)

in Kingston, Usain not only became the youngest ever male gold medallist at the World Junior Championships, but he secured two silver medals while competing for Jamaica in the 4 × 100-metre and the

4 × 400-metre relays. He was coached at William Knibb High School by Olympian Pablo McNeil, the physical education teachers Sheila Thorpe and Dwight Barnett, and an excellent cadre of officials out in Trelawny.

It is no surprise that he emerged out of Boys' Championships to become the only man in the history of the Olympics to set three world records: 9.69 in the 100 metres, 19.30 in the 200 metres and running the third leg on Jamaica's world-record-winning 4 × 100-metre team, that did 37.10 seconds.

Asafa Powell, while not being one of the leading lights at Boys' Championships, was spotted by his coach, Stephen Francis, while competing for Charlemont High School in St Catherine, and, in fact, reached a final at Boys' Championships.

VC: What is so special about Boys' and Girls' Champs that explains why our athletes perform so well on the big stages?

BF: I think it is something about the Champs. It is not often that you perform before, some say, twenty-five thousand people (my understanding of the National Stadium is that when it is full to capacity it can hold thirty-five thousand persons). To have thirty-five thousand persons screaming in a passionate way at your level at your performance must have an indelible impact on your life.

In other words, because, in fact, in 1990 while being a commentator for Jamaica's then-oldest radio station, RJR, I shared the microphones with the late Dr Lennox "Billy" Miller and Linford Christie, the 1992 Olympic 100-metre gold medallist. Christie said that he had never seen anything like that in his life time, and he wished that he could ship that crowd which he saw on the Saturday of the 1990 Boys' Championships to Britain. The National Stadium was absolutely full at capacity of thirty-five thousand. I don't think it can be any better than that.

Christie said he had to go and meet, I don't know if it was with Mr Edward Seaga, but he was going to come late and I said to him "Linford, is one man can save you, so you can get back into the Stadium, and his name is Headley Forbes. . . . I am going to let you meet him and when you are coming, you are to remember the name, head of security, Headley Forbes, or you won't get in." When he did that, he got in, within three minutes, because Mr Forbes took him inside, and when he saw the stadium by then packed beyond capacity, he went like this. [Bobby holding his head (indicating) to Vilma.]

So, in other words, whereas Jamaica has produced Jamaican-born winners for three consecutive Olympic Games, 1988 to 1996, it was not until Bolt in 2008, when we had our very first Jamaican gold medallist in the Olympic 100 metres. In brackets now, we can say the infamous Ben Johnson crossed the line first in 1988, while wearing Canadian colours. He was from Trelawny but he did not compete at Boys' Champs.

Linford Christie, who was the 1992 Jamaican-born Olympic gold medallist in the 100 metres, competed for Britain in the 1992 Olympic Games in Barcelona, Spain. In 1996 it was another Jamaican-born athlete, Donovan Bailey, competing for Canada, who won the Olympic 100 metres in world record time. Donovan had competed in the early years at Boys' Championships, but did not make a significant impact.

Maurice Wignal, while not getting a medal, placed a very commendable fourth place in the 110-metre hurdles in the 2004 Olympic Games in Athens, Greece.

Winthrop Graham, the 1992 Jamaican sportsman of the year, competed for St Elizabeth Technical High School and won gold for them in his specialty, the 400-metre hurdles. He was the 1992 silver medallist at the

Olympic Games in Barcelona, Spain, having beaten the eventual gold medallist, Kevin Young of the United States, in the semifinal, although Young was to go on to set a world record of 46.78 seconds in the final.

Winthrop also won an Olympic silver medal in the 4 × 400 metres, being part of the team comprised of Bertland Cameron, which got silver in 1988 in Seoul, South Korea. Winthrop also has individual bronze and silver medals at the World Championship level.

Recapping, then: with the restart of Girls' Championships in 1957, the women gradually came into their own, and, in fact, there was a period in the 1980s, going into the 1990s, where the female's aspect of the programme was outstripping the boys. The merger of Girls' and Boys' Championships came in the year 1998, and since then Jamaica has been competing with distinction at the highest levels at both the junior, the Olympic and the World Championship levels.

The decision by the relevant authorities to merge the Championships and to ensure that the girls, excellent as they were performing, no longer had to compete before sparse and barren audiences, is now bearing significant fruit. What happened was the girls used to perform in front of a small audience. Like, in that period with Gillian and Nikole, the girls would be doing well but when you go to Girls' Champs it was two thousand, at the most four thousand, spectators. With the merger, the girls also get the strong feeling of being on the stage, and so although not all of them have gone on, we have had instances such as with Aneisha McLaughlin of Holmwood Technical, who has twice won silver in the World Junior Championships in her pet event, the 200 metres, but has not excelled at the senior level. Many unnamed have faced the same obstacles as Aneisha.

VC: Can we just say thanks to Herb McKenley for his contribution?

BF: The late, great Herb McKenley was, during the 1950s, national coach for Jamaica and even up until the 1990s he was still producing and guiding athletes, especially at the junior level, to make sure that the efforts in which he, and Drs George Rhoden and Arthur Wint, started the ball rolling at the Olympic Games of 1948, and also more particularly, Helsinki 1952 were carried on. We can make the point that in 1948, in London in the 400 metres, the gold medallist Arthur Wint was a Calabar High School alumnus, and so was the silver medallist, Herb McKenley.

In 1952, Herb McKenley was suffering from mumps just before the Olympic Games and had entered the 100 metres just to test his fitness, and came within a whisker of winning the gold medal, eventually getting silver. He placed second to his teammate George Rhoden, who won the 1952 Olympic gold medal.

Arthur Wint, Leslie Laing, Herb McKenley and George Rhoden set a world record of 3:03.9 for the 4 × 400-metre relay in the Olympic Games of 1952, shattering the world record by 4.03 seconds. Three of them definitely competed in the Boys' Athletic Championships.

VC: Your concluding thoughts?

BF: The concluding thoughts. Whereas there will be other specific fields which will point to the biochemical and genetic aspects, we must remember that these athletes by having competed before wide and diverse audiences for the past one hundred years, have been tested in the crucible of public domain and have not been found wanting by any stretch of the imagination.

SECTION 5

Protection Issues

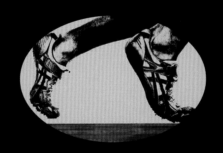

C H A P T E R   1 4

Blood Doping in Sports and Detection Strategies

D O N O V A N   A .   M c G R O W D E R

One of the most serious problems of present-day competitive sports is the increasing usage of various performance-enhancing substances. Doping in various forms has always been a major problem in competitive sports. The first recorded case of using substances enhancing athletes' physical performance dates back to the Olympic Games in the third century BC. The first banned substances were of natural origin and included a beverage made from donkey hooves or dried figs. In the nineteenth century, long-distance swimmers and cyclists were reported to have used performance-enhancing substances such as caffeine, strychnine, ether, alcohol or oxygen. The state of knowledge of human physiology and the effects of different substances on the metabolism of human cells was fairly limited at that time and athletes' abuse of the compounds mentioned led sometimes to their deaths. The first recorded lethal case was cyclist Arthur Linton

who died in 1896 after having taken strychnine (Katarzyne and Gozdzicka-Jozefiak 2008). The absence of drug tests made many athletes enhance their performance with impunity. Taking stimulants, however, did not always yield favourable results and often led to serious health problems. The development of medicine and molecular biology made it possible to use doping adjusted to individual physiological parameters important for a given sport. The number of athletes ready to violate the rules of fair play to achieve better results increases constantly. Many of them are ready to risk their health or even life to take first place.

Rumours that various types of blood doping were being used by athletes to enhance performance began approximately thirty years ago. Blood doping has been the most significant doping problem in endurance sports over the last twenty years. It afforded the greatest performance benefit and has been the most difficult to detect. The definition of blood doping was introduced in the 1970s to describe the use of blood transfusion to increase red cell mass artificially. This allows a higher disposition in oxygen delivery, particularly in sports requiring resistance where aerobic muscular exercise prevails, such as cycling, cross-country skiing, long-distance racing, marathon and triathlon among others (Guezennec 2001). According to the World Anti-Doping Agency (WADA), blood doping is the misuse of certain techniques or substances to increase a person's red blood cell mass, which allows the body to transport more oxygen to muscles and therefore increase stamina and performance. Blood doping was formally added to the list of forbidden methods of enhancing performance in 1985 after many US cyclists admitted having doped themselves with blood during the 1984 Los Angeles Olympic Games. To test for doping, however, a blood sample is required and, over time, legal, ethical and religious issues have hampered blood sampling, as blood collection is an invasive method. Nonetheless, regular tests using blood were performed in athletic competitions in 1993 and 1994. At that time, attention was focused on tracking doping from blood transfusion, in detecting some forbidden endogenous steroids and peptide hormones. For the latter, however, the assays were of very low sensitivity and were done with the use of immunologic techniques.

Jamaica has a proud sprinting tradition at the Olympics which has been firmly established over the past sixty years. At the Olympic Games in Beijing, China, Jamaican athletes won six gold medals, three silver and two bronze. Modern athletics has been overshadowed by doping scandals, and Jamaican athletes are not free of suspicion. In the past, a few Jamaican athletes have tested positive for banned substances. These include nandrolone (19-nortestosterone), bolde-none (1,4-androstadiene-3-one-17β-ol, available as the undecylenate ester), testosterone and salbutamol. Jamaican athletes are tested regularly by the International Association of Athletics Federation (IAAF). In 2008, the IAAF carried out 3,487 anti-doping tests, including scans for the blood booster erythropoietin (EPO), with over half (1,823) taking place out of competition. These figures do not include tests conducted by the International Olympic Committee (IOC) at, or before, the Beijing Games. Jamaica was included in the top five tested nations for the 2008 Olympic season, along with four other countries, namely, Russia, Belarus, the United States and China. The Jamaica Anti-Doping Commission (JADCO) was formed in 2005 to execute the national anti-doping programme in accordance with the international governing body, the WADA. On 10 February 2004, Jamaica became the ninety-seventh signatory state to the UNESCO Copenhagen Declaration on anti-doping in sports and operates under the universal World Anti-Doping Code. Jamaica did not join the Caribbean's Regional Anti-Doping Organisation (RADO) and was criticized for not doing so, particularly with the delay in setting up its own anti-doping body. It was felt that, with Jamaica possessing so many high-calibre international athletes, substantially more than the other Caribbean islands, it merited the country's having its own independent anti-doping body. On 25 July 2008, the Jamaican government approved the Anti-Doping in Sport Act. This is a set of rules which has now become law and will guide all local athletes in relation to doping in sports. The act provides a legal framework to govern doping violations and, thus, to ensure fair play in sports. Since the approval of the act, JADCO has been busy doing preliminary work to manage Jamaica's anti-doping programme effectively. The anti-doping programme will cover all athletes, irrespective of sporting discipline. The process of sample collection has commenced. Athletes will be tested in and out of competition and, in addition, target testing will be done (*Gleaner*, 4 October 2008).

Erythropoietin

Increasing oxygen delivery to tissues is important to optimize muscular activity and improve athletic performance, particularly in terms of endurance. Several methods have been shown to increase oxygen delivery to tissues, including altitude and hypoxic rooms, blood transfusion and treatment with EPO. Erythropoietin represents, for some athletes, the ultimate tool to gain an edge over their peers in competition. It is a 165-amino acid (304 kilodaltons) glycoprotein hormone produced mainly in the kidneys, in the liver (< 10 per cent) and in very little quantities in the brain. The carbohydrate content of EPO is about 40 per cent, and like other plasma glycoproteins, EPO circulates in a pool of isoforms that differ in glycosylation and biological activity. Erythropoietin is the main regulator of erythropoiesis (production of red blood cells) and the physiological stimulus for EPO production is tissue hypoxia (low oxygen) which, in most instances, is directly related to the number of circulating erythrocytes (red blood cells). Thus, EPO and erythropoiesis are part of a negative feedback cycle that keeps tissue oxygen delivery within a narrow range by controlling the number of erythrocytes circulating in the blood (Donnelly 2001).

In a normal individual, any loss of red blood cells due to bleeding or haemolysis decreases the delivery of oxygen to the tissues. When low oxygen in the tissue is sensed by cells in the kidney and liver capable of pro-

ducing EPO, these cells then produce and secrete EPO into the plasma. The EPO is carried to the bone marrow, where it binds to specific cell surface receptors on its target cells (Miller, Heilman and Wojchowski 2002). The binding of EPO by these cells increases their ability to survive and reach the reticulocyte stage, and thereby contribute to the population of circulating red blood cells. The increased numbers of circulating red blood cells in turn deliver more oxygen to the tissues. This increased oxygen delivery is sensed by the EPO-producing cells which then reduce EPO production so that the normal steady-state number of red blood cells is restored. Depending on the sports modality, EPO administration to elite athletes may lead to an artificial performance improvement, decreasing, for instance, their time marks. So, in order to maintain the health of the individual and sports ethics, the IOC and other sports federations considered the use of EPO and its analogue drugs as blood-doping cases. The use of EPO was banned in sports by the IOC in 1987.

Recombinant EPO (rHuEPO)

Availability of this class of compounds in the market dramatically increased in the 1980s, with the advent of recombinant deoxyribonucleic acid (DNA) technology. The synthetic form of EPO, recombinant human EPO (rHuEPO), was genetically engineered for therapeutic use in 1987 and marketing began in 1988. Since then, it has been successfully used in medical care. It has improved the quality of life of patients in constant need of blood transfusions, or with anaemia due to chronic renal failure. Several types of rHuEPO are commercially available, including Epoetin alpha (Eprex, Janssen-Cilag), Epoetin beta (Neorecormon, Roche) and Darbepoetin alpha (Nespo, Dompè) (Caldini et al. 2003). The recombinant forms of EPO have indiscriminately been used by athletes, mainly in endurance sports, to increase the erythrocyte concentration, thereby generating a better delivery of oxygen to the muscle tissue. It may have been used as early as 1988 in the Calgary Winter Olympics skiing events.

Recombinant EPO is a glycoprotein of 304 kDa. It has a short half-life, although its effects in the blood only become evident 3 to 5 days after administration. These effects subsist for one to several weeks in cases of prolonged treatment. If treatment is stopped a few days before competition, the athlete thus benefits from its effects without risk of its being detected. After intravenous administration, maximum serum rHuEPO concentration peaks are reached within minutes, whereas time to reach maximum peak values from subcutaneous administration may range from 5 to 24 hours after administration, or a little more (Goldberg 1995). Clinical trials carried out in the mid 1990s to assess intravenous and subcutaneous routes of administration did not show differences in the effectiveness of treatment or in blood pressure when the two routes were compared.

Immediately after rHuEPO became available as an erythropoiesis-stimulating drug, it was reputed to be abused by athletes in aerobic sports. Recombinant EPO doping by healthy athletes who do not need any treatment is not acceptable and the risk of developing disease is potential, and may lead to dependence on continuing blood transfusions for the rest of their lives. Fatal cases connected to doping occurred in the early 1990s, when professional Dutch cyclists competing in Europe died at rest, some of them while sleeping, due to unexplainable cardiac arrest (Cazzola 2002). These sportsmen are among the more than twenty cases of

deaths of cyclists in Europe reported between 1987 and 1991, when rHuEPO was first made available in that continent (Gareau et al. 1996). Evidence on the use of rHuEPO was found after a blood check of Italian professional cyclists showed serum iron overloads comparable to those of genetic haemochromatose patients. The levels of ferritin (a protein associated with the amount of iron stored in the body) in these cyclists were abnormally high, a clear sign of intravenous iron and rHuEPO administration (Cazzola 2002). In 1989, the IOC Medical Commission introduced the new doping class of peptide hormones and analogues, which includes rHuEPO, human chorionic gonadotrophin and related compounds, adrenocorticotrophic hormone, human growth hormone and all the releasing factors of these hormones which are required for their synthesis.

In 1998, discovering rHuEPO ampoules with cyclists of a number of teams participating in the Tour de France was probably the most striking and publicized case pf rHuEPO doping in recent sporting events. At the time, boxes with many ampoules of the drug were found in trucks of the main participating teams and even in the competitors' lodgings, reflecting endemic use of this hormone among elite athletes. Over the twenty-one days of competition drug busts, enquiries and arrests were part of the competitions, which French newspapers called "Tour de Farce". Some athletes, after developing health problems from the illicit use of rHuEPO, admitted having used this hormone (Jarvis 1999). Such is the case of a cyclist who presented with strong headache, nausea, vomiting and photophobia two months before a competition. He was diagnosed with idiopathic intracranial hypertension, non-responsive to standard treatment. Medical examination and laboratory tests suggested the use of rHuEPO, which was confirmed by the athlete upon questioning (Lage et al. 2002). In spite of all the above cases, liberation of the drug has been advocated by some groups. They argue that because rHuEPO is impossible to be detected, it is best to allow its use. The IOC, however, has included this recombinant hormone in the roll of forbidden drugs since 1990, after the Calgary Winter Games, where its use was evidenced, and the Seoul Olympic Games. Such prohibition was just on a moral ground, due to lack of technology to fully detect and differentiate rHuEPO from endogenous EPO.

The main risks of erythrocytosis include heart failure, myocardial infarction, seizures, peripheral thromboembolic events and pulmonary embolism. The risks are raised during competition when blood viscosity increases further due to intensified perspiration and the shift of fluid from the intravascular into the interstitial space (Szygula 1990). The fact that the above-mentioned cases of the deaths of cyclists suspected of rHuEPO doping did not occur during exercise but during periods of physical inactivity does not militate against the detrimental effect of erythrocytosis. Blood flow in microcirculation slows down during physical inactivity, thereby favouring the development of thrombi. The risk of EPO's promoting tumour growth has been considered (Tentori and Graziani 2007), although supporting clinical evidence is missing.

Detecting Misuse in Sports

In 1997, the International Union of Cyclists (IUC) implemented random blood tests before each competition. These tests involved measuring the level of haematocrit and ruled that male athletes with a reading value of more than 50 per cent and female athletes with haematocrit higher than 47 per cent could not compete because the competition would be hazardous for them (Ekblom and Berglund 1991). The IUC stated that the tests performed were health assessments to prevent athletes with a "dangerously high" haematocrit from competing. A positive test result does not necessarily imply rHuEPO use, and therefore athletes were suspended for two weeks only. Haematocrit is a physiological variable closely related to performance enhancement in exercise. An investigation carried out with the subcutaneous administration of rHuEPO has shown increased haematocrit, elevated maximum oxygen intake and systolic blood pressure and extended time of exhaustion from exercise. The side effects described for rHuEPO are more marked when excessive hormone doses raise haematocrit to values between 50 and 55 per cent, which typically occurs with endurance sports due to natural dehydration (Wadler 1994). The IUC subsequently adopted as an additional criterion for allowing athletes to compete the maximum level of 17g/dL for serum haemoglobin (Cazzola 2002). The International Federation of Ski also implemented banning procedures for athletes, and adopted the limit of 18.5 g/dL for serum haemoglobin.

There were controversies on the imposed upper limit of haemocrit. Limitation factors included dehydration status, the hour of the day the sample is drawn, large natural variation between individuals, risk of false positivity, ease of manipulation through interventions such as saline infusion, and the posture of the athlete. There are a small number of elite athletes with naturally high haematocrit values. The latter has been rebutted by the fact that haematocrit values from blood samples of athletes who competed before rHuEPO became available in the market were within the specified limits. Excessively high limit values of haemocrit only result in more doping tests, fostering athletes to take rHuEPO with the aim of approaching the target haematocrit or haemoglobin without exceeding it (which is possible with the extended use of low doses of hormone). Portable cell counters and centrifuges to ensure the established limits were not exceeded were ever-present tools in sports arena.

Indirect Methods for Detecting EPO

The availability of rHuEPO in 1987 in Europe made it possible to use ergogenic hormones illicitly in endurance sports. Two philosophies were developed for the detection of rHuEPO misuse in sports. The first one was based on the detection of indirect blood markers, and the second was based on the direct detection of rHuEPO in urine (Breymann 2000). The promotion of secondary blood markers was mainly on the basis that they could be used to detect rHuEPO injected a long time ago (more than a week) and also that these markers could be used to detect erythropoietic stimulators such as erythropoietin alpha, beta, omega and delta, darbepoetin alpha and mimetic peptides (Johnson and Jolliffe 2000). Furthermore, secondary blood markers could eventually be used to identify athletes who ceased using rHuEPO or other erythropoietic stimulators. The direct detection of rHuEPO in blood or urine has the advantage of identifying the drug itself (or metabolites), but had the disadvantage of being expensive, insensitive and difficult to perform.

In the last ten years, a number of studies have investigated indirect methods for the detection of rHuEPO abuse by means of parameters indicative of accelerated erythropoiesis. Parameters closely related to rHuEPO administration include haematocrit (Hct), reticulocyte Hct (retHct), percentage of macrocytes, soluble trans-ferring receptor (sTfR) and serum EPO. These parameters were then utilized to develop mathematical models aimed at discriminating between athletes given rHuEPO and those given placebo. Two models were developed based on the behaviour of each of the five parameters during and after controlled treatment with rHuEPO (Parisotto et al. 2003). The "ON" model is applied during or shortly after rHuEPO treatment, whereas the "OFF" model is used weeks after termination of treatment (Kazlauskas, Howe and Trout 2002). A simpler approach employs only a combination of haemoglobin level, concentration of serum EPO and percentage of reticulocytes; it was found to have higher sensitivity in cases of low dose rHuEPO abuse (Pascual et al. 2004). It was found that the ON model repeatedly identified 94 to 100 per cent of rHuEPO group members during the final two weeks of the rHuEPO administration phase (one false positive from a possible 189), while the OFF model repeatedly identified 67 to 72 per cent of recent users with no false positives (Parisotto et al. 2000). If these parameters were unusual, isoelectric focusing (IEF) of urine samples was then employed to provide proof of rHuEPO abuse (Wilber 2002). The combination of the blood parameters with urine IEF was approved by the IOC in 2001. This test resulted in the forfeiture of medals won by three cross-country skiers in the Salt Lake City Winter Olympics in 2002 (De Frutos, Cifuentes and Diez-Masa 2003).

All parameters involved in the previous equations except retHct were known to be affected by changes in erythropoiesis. However, some drawbacks to these models were associated with the dependency of some of the parameters on cellular volume, potentially affected by blood storage and transportation conditions. Consequently, a second generation of models with higher robustness that were simpler to apply were proposed

(Gore et al. 2003). The new equations used concentrations of haemoglobin ([Hb]), EPO and sTfR as well as percentage reticulocytes when compared with the total number of erythrocytes. The two new equations were labelled ON he and ON hr. Some sports authorities (for example, Australian Sports Drug Agency) have used longitudinal studies with these models for early alerting to some abnormality related to the production of erythrocytes.

Although immunoassays are of little use in direct detection of recombinant protein abuse, they play an essential role in the determination of the indirect markers of rHuEPO abuse. Different immunoassays can be used for the determination of serum EPO and STfR concentrations (Abellan et al. 2004). Potential for a greater role of immunoassays in the detection process is generated by the production of a monoclonal antibody against rHuEPO. Sample integrity issues may pose additional complications in the detection of recombinant proteins. For example, there is a need to protect EPO against proteases in urine samples used in IEF. Another problem is presented by the time and temperature dependence of blood samples to be analysed for rHuEPO abuse. Such samples have to be analysed as soon as possible, preferably on the site of the competition to avoid the decline of red blood cell analytes with time and temperature. Reticulocyte percentage and haematocrit level (reliable only for a few hours) were found to be vulnerable (Robinson, Mangin and Saugy 2004). Sample transportation to other testing locations even at low temperatures poses a significant risk of sample analyte deterioration due to mechanical stress. Another important issue to be considered is the effect of haematological abnormalities in the tested athletes which are unrelated to the doping process. However, it was found that most haematological disorders found in top athletes do not lead to values higher than the cut-offs for the rHuEPO model tests; actually, most were found to give lower values. Therefore, the effect of such conditions on rHuEPO testing is mostly negligible (Parisotto et al. 2000).

Direct Methods for Detecting EPO

In the year 2000, there was a major breakthrough in the detection of rHuEPO in human urine. Lasne and Ceaurriz (2000) reported a direct test to detect rHuEPO based on subtle differences between rHuEPO and physiological EPO carbohydrate residues. Isoelectric focusing detects the presence of rHuEPO in the urine (uEPO) and constitutes a major improvement both in the resolution of the isoforms (the electrophoretic bands) and in its sensitivity. Disposition of the bands for rHuEPO alpha and beta forms (epoetina) is very similar (both present isoelectric points ranging from 4.42 to 5.11) even though epoetin beta presents extra basic bands. Both differ from natural, purified EPO (with more acid bands, and isoelectric points ranging from 3.92 to 4.42). This test was assayed before the Sydney Olympic Games, in competitors of the 1998 Tour de France, and showed bands typical of the recombinant hormone in athletes suspected of abusing it (Lasne and Ceaurriz 2000). The data collected at that time showed that urine tests would detect the hormone up to three days after the last rHuEPO injection, which would allow for athletes to keep on using rHuEPO up to few days prior to the competition, thus participating in the event while under the effect of the hormone. This test would, therefore, be more suited to screening athletes in the pre-season or as a complementary test to the indirect test (Zorpette 2000).

Both urine and blood tests for rHuEPO analysis were used at the Sydney Olympic Games in 2000. However, to prevent the possibility of a false positive result, sanctions were only taken with positive results for both tests. At that time, Olympic Committee officials stated that athletes who refused to submit to the tests claiming ethical or moral reasons would be instantly excluded from the competition (Birchard 2000). No positive case for rHuEPO was reported during the Olympics even though there was some indication that a small number of athletes had apparently discontinued the use of rHuEPO a few weeks prior to their arrival in Sydney. Only 400 anti-rHuEPO tests were performed in Sydney in relation to the total number of competitors. This low proportion favoured the user athlete as only one out of twenty athletes was sampled for rHuEPO, and "the idea of one having clean games was nothing other than an utopic fantasy" (Birchard 2000). Since then, rHuEPO analyses based on the described methods were performed in major international sports events, such as the 2002 Winter Games in Salt Lake City. Over the competitions in this event, a total of 1,222 blood tests and a combined 72 blood and urine tests to detect rHuEPO were performed. For this event, 77 blood and urine combined tests were also made outside of competitions. No positive case for rHuEPO was found at that time. However, three positive cases have been described for another synthetic hormone analogue to EPO which has been recently released in the market. It is labelled "darbepoetin alpha". This hormone is a hyperglycosylated EPO analogue that is biochemically different from other rHuEPO forms. It has two additional carbohydrate chains bound to nitrogen atoms, and amino acid replacements in five positions of the peptide skeleton. Darbepoetin fosters production of red cells, thus being capable of enhancing performance of athletes, particu-

larly in endurance sports (Egrie and Browne 2001). It is detected by the IEF method.

At present the IEF method, together with clarifications in the technical document from WADA, forms what is still the only method able to identify the presence of rHuEPO or darbepoetin in the presence of their ubiquitous endogenous counterpart (uEPO). It is considered reliable and valid. Capillary zone electrophoresis also has the potential for the detection of rHuEPO. This technique is based on the different glycosylation patterns between endogenous uEPO and rHuEPO. The main peculiarity of this technique is due to the difference in sialic acid groups (De Frutos, Cifuentes and Diez-Masa 2003).

Growth Hormone

One of the most commonly abused substances in sports over the last decades has undoubtedly been growth hormone, which is also known as somatotrophin. Growth hormone is a protein hormone which is secreted in large pulses from the anterior pituitary. The GH secretion is stimulated during sleep, fever, physical exercise and stress, as well as by some amino acids (leucine, arginine) and hormones (estrogens and androgens). Long and intense physical exercise can elevate GH secretion up to ten times the normal value (Ehrnborg, Bengtsson and Rosen 2000). Somatotrophin has anabolic activity. Its protein synthesis potential is comparable to that of testosterone. Important mediators in GH activity are insulin-like growth factors (IGF-I, IGF-II) synthesized in the liver stimulated by GH. In 1989, recombinant human growth hormone (rhGH) was developed. The rhGH treatment of patients with GH deficiency increases muscle mass and lean body mass, reduces adipose tissue and enhances the functioning of the heart and kidneys (Ehrnborg, Bengtsson and Rosen 2000). Growth hormone became commercially available as an ergogenic aid in 1988 and soon became immensely popular among athletes who were interested in the enhancement of their training quality. The attractiveness to GH relied on a conviction that the hormone strengthens tendons, accelerates tissue regeneration, increases muscle mass, and strengthens and reduces the fat deposition. Its main advantages were anabolic activity, accessibility, small risk of side effects and impossibility to detect (Sonksen 2001).

Growth hormone is mainly abused by athletes in strength-based sports, sprinters as well as endurance sports athletes and soccer players. It is often used by women as it entails no risk of androgenic side effects (Ehrnborg, Bengtsson and Rosen 2000). A number of outstanding athletes were known to use GH doping. Ben Johnson was stripped of his Olympic gold medal from Seoul in 1988 after having admitted taking GH in combination with anaerobic steroids for many years (Sonksen 2001). Despite the conviction about the absolute safety of GH use, there are indications that a long-term administration can increase the risk of diabetes mellitus, retention of fluids, joint and muscle pain, hypertension, cardiomyopathy, osteoporosis, irregular menstruation and impotence (Humbel 1990).

The inherent features of hGH made the detection of rhGH an even more troublesome endeavour than that of rHuEPO. Human GH has a short half life (< 15 min) and exists in urine samples at very low concentrations. As a result, urine samples cannot be used for testing. One approach is based on the use of immunoassays for the detection of different isoforms of endogenous hGH (Bidlingmaier, Wu and Strasburger 2003). Recombinant hGH consists only of one isoform which is 22 kDa,

whereas the endogenous hGH consists of different isoforms of various sizes. Administration of rhGH (22 kDa) will repress pituitary secretion of hGH by negative feedback. Thus, if immunoassay analysis of serum shows abnormally elevated levels of the 22 kDa protein, this would indicate illegal use of rhGH (Bidlingmaier, Wu and Strasburger 2003). Another approach avoids detection of hGH protein itself; instead, it focuses on the pharmacodynamic endpoints of hGH action such as changes in parameters modulated by hGH. Human GH exerts most of its functions through the generation of IGF-I. In one study, treatment of athletes ($n = 15$) with 0.06 IU hGH/kg/day for fourteen days resulted in a rapid increase in IGF-I concentrations even three days after initiation of treatment (Kniess et al. 2003). It has been suggested that hGH abusers may take up to 25 IU/day, which is much higher than the dose of 1–2 IU/day given to GH-deficient patients (Bidlingmaier, Wu and Strasburger 2003). Both hGH and its mediator, IGF-I, are potent mitogenic and anti-apoptotic agents, and several reports have shown an association between IGF-I levels and the incidence of breast, prostate and colorectal cancers (Allen et al. 2005).

Gene Doping

The field of gene therapy is evolving and may soon open the door for a more insidious doping method termed "gene doping". The aim of gene doping is to produce recombinant proteins within human cells, rather than introducing the recombinant product into the body. In the 2005 prohibited list published by the WADA, gene doping is defined as the "non-therapeutic use of cells, genes, genetic elements, or modulation of gene expression, having the capacity to enhance athletic performance". The list of prohibited substances tested for gene doping becomes longer each year. The most popular substances include growth hormone (GH), erythropoietin (EPO), insulin, IFG-I, haemoglobin-based oxygen carriers (HBCOs), alpha-actinin 3 (ACTN3), angiotensin convertase (ACE), hypoxia inducible factor (HIF-1α), delta peroxisome proliferative activated receptor delta (PPAR), and endothelial growth factor (VEGF).

Gene doping stemmed out of the legitimate gene therapy experiments which are based on strategies for treating genetic diseases by introducing and expressing a deficient gene or by modulating the activity of an existing gene (Unal and Ozer Unal 2004). In vivo introduction of the target (artificial) gene into the human genome can be achieved by biological (viral vectors), physical (direct injection using a syringe or gene gun) or chemical methods. Ex vivo gene doping can include gene transfer to cells in culture and re-introduction of the genetically modified cells into the host. Gene therapy or doping using viral vectors is the most efficient method in which replication deficient vectors derived from retroviruses, adenoviruses or lentiviruses are used to deliver the gene of interest. The genetically engineered viruses are then introduced into the body, where they infect the cells and recruit the cells' biochemical machinery to express the transgene. Such vectors offer several advantages of long-term expression, low anti-vector immunity, cell-specific tropism and large packaging capacity (Sinn, Sauter and McCray 2005). However, it should be noted that integrating gene transfer vectors poses a risk of insertional mutagenesis (Sinn, Sauter and McCray 2005).

A number of conceptual and practical factors have led to the fact that no tests are currently available to detect gene doping. The protein produced by the foreign gene or genetically manipulated cells will be identical to the endogenous one. Most gene doping proteins, particularly muscle enhancing ones, are generated locally in the muscle and do not show in blood or urine, as is the case with IGF-I. The only reliable assay would require a muscle biopsy, which is inapplicable in a sports setting.

Technical challenges are not the only obstacles facing detection efforts. There are cost-related issues that could become a major limitation to anti-doping efforts. Doping prevention efforts, from basic research and development of new diagnostic strategies to the awareness and coordination of programmes, are extremely costly. The fight against doping also involves huge educational, awareness and monitoring projects, which fall within WADA's scope of activities. Research involving detection of recombinant proteins and gene doping constitutes at least three of WADA's four priority research themes. The increasing threat of gene doping and recombinant proteins can be expected to have a dramatic impact on the sample volume to be tested at major sports events. The capacity, speed and technologies of anti-doping laboratories are improving, but so are the numbers of athletes and the demand for stricter doping control in competitive sports. The most difficult challenge may be the logistics involved in coordinating the various international authorities and athletes for education about doping. These challenges extend to corporations involved in producing recombinant proteins. It is difficult to estimate accurately the total cost of doping control; however, this complicated issue must be navigated carefully because it extends far beyond scientific excellence and athletic dedication. In any case, WADA appears to have little choice except to take an aggressive and comprehensive stance because the integrity of sporting competition is at stake.

Future Perspectives

In their work on the reappraisal of the abuse of drugs by athletes, Duntas and Parisis have cited the ancient Greek saying "none so wretched as the competitor who wins through cheating". Yet the authors have conceded that commercialization has progressively changed the spirit of the sport, as the desire to win at any cost has overcome all ethical and medical considerations. Success in elite sports gives promise of fame and financial rewards. Moreover, trainers and sports officials press their protégés for victories and spectators long for heroes.

As the recombinant DNA technology advances, the potential of doping methods increases. The quality of recombinant proteins used is likely to improve. With several novel erythropoietic drugs on the market, doping control has become very difficult, not to say hopeless. The new drugs include various kinds of epoetins, biosimilars, mutated EPO analogues, long-acting pegylated epoetins and EPO analogues, EPO fusion proteins, and peptidic as well as non-peptidic EPO mimetics. Compounds are at hand which act as stabilizers of hypoxia-inducible transcription factors (HIF) that bind to the EPO enhancer. Because EPO signalling involves protein tyrosine phosphorylation, inhibitors of haemopoietic cell phosphatase (HCP) may also become available for misuse (Barbone et al. 1999). The novel drugs are being developed primarily for therapeutic benefits, that is, the alleviation of anaemia in patients suffering from chronic renal failure or inflammatory or malignant diseases. The detection of these drugs will become even more challenging. At the same time, the appeal of the doping method and the increasingly lucrative nature of competitive sports make the situation even more difficult. This puts increasing pressure on clinical scientists to develop reliable and practical methods for its detection, alongside keeping up with the current notorious substance doping using recombinant proteins. Although the concepts of efficient detection are practically fully developed, the actual challenge lies in resolving the technical aspects of the detection methods. These include pre-analytical variables such as vigorous exercise, storage conditions, and time elapsed for samples to reach the anti-doping laboratories. It should be noted that most athletes may not have enough background to comprehend fully the potential risks imposed by gene doping. Therefore, educating athletes as well as their supporting staff would be crucial in minimizing both the abuse of recombinant proteins and gene doping. One can sum up the current challenge in the following way: How can one practically differentiate among substances that have the same structure, do the same job in the same place? This is the exact question sports clinical chemists are trying to answer at the moment. In addition, because there are not only major technical problems in detecting the drugs for proof of doping but also difficulties with respect to intention, moral and law, it is crucial to inform athletes and their supporting staff of potential health risks, although this may be an act of "throwing caution to the wind".

References

Abellan, R., R. Ventura, S. Pichini, A.F. Remacha, J.A. Pascual, R. Pacifici et al. 2004. Evaluation of immunoassays for the measurement of erythropoietin (EPO) as an indirect biomarker of recombinant human EPO misuse in sport. *Journal of Pharmaceutical and Biomedical Analysis* 35:1169–77.

Allen, N.E., A.W. Roddam, D.S. Allen, I.S. Fentiman, I. Dos Santos Silva, J. Peto et al. 2005. A prospective study of serum insulin-like growth factor-I (IGF-I), IGF-II, IGF-binding protein-3 and breast cancer risk. *British Journal of Cancer* 92:1283–87.

Barbone, F.P., D.L. Johnson, F.X. Farrell, A. Collins, S.A. Middleton, F.J. McMahon et al. 1999. New epoetin molecules and novel therapeutic approaches. *Nephrology, Dialysis, Transplantation* 14:80–84.

Bidlingmaier, M., Z. Wu and C.J. Strasburger. 2003. Problems with GH doping in sports. *Journal of Endocrinological Investigation* 26:924–31.

Birchard, K. 2000. Past, present, and future of drug abuse at the Olympics. *Lancet* 356:1008.

Breymann, C. 2000. Erythropoietin test methods. *Best Practice and Research Clinical Endocrinology and Metabolism* 14:135–45.

Caldini, A., G. Moneti, A. Fanelli, A. Bruschettini, S. Mercurio, G. Pieraccini et al. 2003. Epoetin alpha, epoetin beta and darbepoetin alfa: two-dimensional gel electrophoresis isoforms characterization and mass spectrometry analysis. *Proteomics* 3:937–41.

Cazzola, M. 2002. A global strategy for prevention and detection of blood doping with erythropoietin and related drugs. *Haematologica* 85:561–63.

De Frutos, M., A. Cifuentes and J.C. Diez-Masa. 2003. Differences in capillary electrophoresis profiles of urinary and recombinant erythropoietin. *Electrophoresis* 24:678–80.

Donnelly, S. 2001. Why is erythropoietin made in the kidney? The kidney functions as a critmeter. *American Journal of Kidney Diseases* 38:415–25.

Egrie, J.C., and J.K. Browne. 2001. Development and characterization of novel erythropoiesis stimulating protein (NESP). *British Journal of Cancer* 84:3–10.

Ehrnborg, C., B-A. Bengtsson and T. Rosen. 2000. Growth hormone abuse. *Best Practice and Research Clinical Endocrinology and Metabolism* 14:71–77.

Ekblom, B., and B. Berglund. 1991. Effect of erythropoietin administration on maximal aerobic power. *Scandinavian Journal of Medicine and Science in Sports* 1:88–93.

Gareau, R., M. Audran, R.D. Baynes, C.H. Flowers, A. Duvallet, L. Senécal et al. 1996. Erythropoietin abuse in athletes. *Nature* 380:113.

Goldberg, M.A. 1995. Erythropoiesis, erytropoietin, and iron metabolism in selective surgery: Preoperative strategies for avoiding allogeneic blood exposure. *American Journal of Surgery* 179: S37–43.

Gore, C.J., R. Parisotto, M.J. Ashenden, J. Stray-Gundersen, K. Sharpe, W. Hopkins, K.R. Emslie, C. Howe, G.J. Trout, R. Kazlauskas and A.G. Hahn. 2003. Second-generation blood tests to detect erythropoietin abuse by athletes. *Haematologica* 88:333–44.

Guezennec, Ch-Y. 2001. Le dopage: Efficacité, conséquences, prévention. *Annales d'endocrinologie* 62:33–41.

Humbel, R.E. 1990. Insulin-like growth factors I and II. *European Journal of Biochemistry* 190 (3): 445–62.

Jarvis, C.A. 1999. Tour de France. *British Journal of Sports Medicine* 33:142–43.

Johnson, D.L., and L.K. Jolliffe. 2000. Erythropoietin mimetic peptides and the future. *Nephrology, Dialysis, Transplantation* 15:1274–77.

Katarzyne, K., and A. Gozdzicka-Jozefiak. 2008. Doping in sports: New development. *Human Movement* 9 (1): 62–75.

Kazlauskas, R., C. Howe and G. Trout. 2002. Strategies for rhEPO detection in sport. *Clinical Journal of Sport Medicine* 12:229–35.

Kniess, A., E. Ziegler, J. Kratzsch, D. Thieme, R.K. Muller.

2003. Potential parameters for the detection of hGH doping. *Analytical and Bioanalytical Chemistry* 376:696–700.

Lage, J.M.M., C. Panizo, J. Masdeu and E. Rocha. 2002. Cyclist's doping associated with cerebral sinus thrombosis. *Neurology* 58:665.

Lasne, F., and J. de Ceaurriz. 2000. Recombinant erythropoietin in urine. *Nature* 405:635.

Miller, C.P., D.W. Heilman and D.M. Wojchowski. 2002. Erythropoietin receptor-dependent erythroid colony-forming unit development: Capacities of Y343 and phosphotyrosine-null receptor forms. *Blood* 99:898–904.

Parisotto, R., M.J. Ashenden, C.J. Gore, K. Sharpe, W. Hopkins and A.G. Hahn. 2003. The effect of common hematologic abnormalities on the ability of blood models to detect erythropoietin abuse by athletes. *Haematologica* 88:931–40.

Parisotto, R., C.J. Gore, K.R. Emslie, M.J. Ashenden, C. Brugnara, C. Howe et al. 2000. A novel method utilizing markers of altered erythropoiesis for the detection of recombinant human erythropoietin abuse in athletes. *Haematologica* 85:564–72.

Pascual, J.A., V. Belalcazar, C. de Bolos, R. Gutierrez, E. Llop and J. Segura. 2004. Recombinant erythropoietin and analogues: A challenge for doping control. *Therapeutic Drug Monitoring* 26:175–79.

Robinson, N., P. Mangin and M. Saugy. 2004. Time and temperature dependant changes in red blood cell analytes used for testing recombinant erythropoietin abuse in sports. *Clinical Laboratory* 50:317–23.

Sinn, P.L., S.L. Sauter and P.B. McCray. 2005. Gene therapy progress and prospects: Development of improved lentiviral and retroviral vectors – Design, biosafety, and production. *Gene Therapy* 12:1089–98.

Sonksen, P.H. 2001. Insulin, growth hormone and sport. *Journal of Endocrinology* 170 (1): 1324–25.

Szygula, Z. 1990. Erythrocytic system under the influence of physical exercise and training. *Sports Medicine* 10:181–97.

Tentori, L., and G. Graziani. 2007. Doping with growth hormone/IGF-1, anabolic steroids or erythropoietin: Is there a cancer risk? *Pharmacological Research* 55 (5): 359–69.

Unal, M., and D. Ozer Unal. 2004. Gene doping in sports. *Sports Medicine* 34:357–62.

Wadler, G.I. 1994. Drug use update. *Sports Medicine* 78:439–55.

Wilber, R.L. 2002. Detection of DNA-recombinant human epoetin- alpha as a pharmacological ergogenic aid. *Sports Medicine* 32:125–42.

Zorpette, G. 2000. All doped up and going for the gold. *Scientific American* 282: 20–22.

CHAPTER 15

Elite Athletes

The Importance of Haematologic Passports

RACHAEL IRVING

According to the World Anti-Doping Agency's (WADA) models of best practice (2008), anti-doping programmes seek to preserve what is intrinsically valuable about sport. An anti-doping rule is violated if a prohibited substance, or its metabolite or marker, is detected in an athlete's sample. It must be noted, however, that a quantitative threshold is specifically identified for certain substances on the prohibited list; therefore, the presence of certain biochemical parameters and metabolites outside of acceptable ranges has the potential to influence the indices of blood doping and the results of anti-doping tests.

A haematologic or blood passport can be used to explain biological variations of blood and urine parameters in professional athletes. Blood and urine samples are repeatedly tested over a specified period. The repeated serial tests are used to define the athlete's specific ranges for various biological substances. A unique medical profile or passport is created from these tests and can be used to challenge or confirm any questionable anti-doping results. Genetic variants in individuals can be noted in a blood passport. Former WADA president Dick Pound reported in 2007 that anti-doping passports may become widespread within three years. Many of the developed countries are at present designing blood passports for their elite athletes.

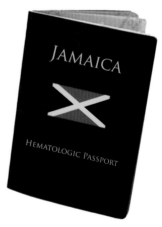

PLATE 15.1 A haematological or blood passport: the new frontier of antidoping testing.

Common Doping Offences

The following are commonly used in doping offences:

1. Anabolic steroids are synthetic drugs that mimic the properties of the male hormone, testosterone. Anabolic steroids may be taken as tablets, as powder or by intramuscular injection to improve muscle growth and power. Anabolic steroids are usually taken in cycles of weeks or months followed by short resting or break periods (cycling). Most of the doping offences related to sprinters are associated with anabolic steroids.

2. Erythropoietin (EPO) is a protein hormone produced by the kidneys. Erythropoietin controls the production of red blood cells, or erythropoiesis. Erythropoietin causes an increase in red blood cell volume, thereby enabling more oxygen to flow to the muscles. The mainly slow-twitch muscles used in endurance running utilize more oxygen than the fast-twitch muscles of sprinters. Recombinant or synthetic EPO is often the illegal drug used to enhance performance in endurance events. Autologous blood transfusion mimics the effects of erythropoietin and can also be used to enhance endurance.

3. Tetrahydrogestrinone (THG), or "clear", is the most potent synthetic steroid to date. This drug was designed to change the genomic profile of cells, thus affecting translation and transcription of certain proteins. The drug couples the benefits of natural aerobic and anaerobic metabolism of muscle cells by inducing an interaction between androgen action and oxygen consumption. This is done by activating a natural metabolic enzyme (bisphosphoglycerate mutase). The chemical synthesis of THG was designed to escape detection since the compound degrades during standard gas chromatography and mass spectrometry procedures (tests used by the WADA-accredited labs to detect illegal substances in samples). The degraded compound is passed out undetectable in the urine. Before this designer compound was sent by an unknown source to the IOC, there was no known test robust enough to detect the substance. Marion Jones is said to have admitted to using "clear" although it was never detected in any of her tested samples.

Natural Occurrences That May Be Classified as Doping Offences

The testosterone/epitestosterone ratio should be < 4.1. Values above the 4.1 ratio might indicate doping; however, high levels of testosterone may be due naturally to the dysregulation of the testicular secretion of epitestosterone (Dehennin 1994). Minor change or polymorphism in the gene (CYP17 promoter) involved in the production of a compound which is a precursor of epitestosterone will also affect the testosterone/epitestosterone ratio, therefore pushing results outside of the acceptable normal range.

Nandrolone is an anabolic steroid that may be present naturally in humans, usually in minute quantities of less than 0.4 ng/ml. Nandrolone can be indirectly detected by testing urine for metabolite 19-norandrosterone. The IOC's acceptable range is < 2.0 ng/ml. It is said that taking in too much lysine causes elevation of nandrolone levels.

Some persons have a mutated version of the gene *EPOR*, which causes increased production of red blood cells. Increased red cells provide more oxygen to muscles and reduce fatigue. Increased red cell volume is usually associated with recombinant erythropoietin (EPO) usage or blood doping. However, this is not always the case, as researchers have identified an entire Finnish family with this *EPOR* mutation, several of whom were championship endurance athletes, including the gold medal cross-country skier Eero Maentyranta.

Taking the So-called Safe Supplements

Supplements are often contaminated with banned substances as there is no strict regulation of this billion-dollar industry. It is reported that 10 to 20 per cent of supplements have hidden ingredients that are not listed on the label, and that these ingredients are sometimes banned steroids. A longitudinal profile or blood passport would indicate changes in natural blood parameters after ingestion of possible contaminated substances. If an athlete is therefore sanctioned based on the strict liability clause after taking a supplement that he or she did not know was contaminated, the athlete has reason to sue the supplier or manufacturer.

Male/Female Determination

Originally, a male is defined as a person having the XY chromosomes and a female the XX chromosomes. There is a term or a problem that is becoming increasingly noticeable, that is, intersex or genital ambiguity, refered to in some societies as the third sex (Agrawal 1997). A person may be born with mosaic genetics, so that some of her cells have XX chromosomes and some XY. Testosterone is linked to speed. A male usually produces more testosterone than a female and goes faster

over a particular distance. It is conceivable that someone with mosaic genetics will have a top speed that is in between that of a male and a female. As scientific knowledge increases and areas once thought clear become blurred, it is imperative that all athletes do a biological profile. In the event that ambiguous areas are questioned, records will show that all legal safeguards were taken in accordance with current standards.

Discrepancies in Laboratory Results

Although EPO misuse in sports is rampant, sometimes WADA-accredited laboratories give conflicting results for samples from the same individual. Lundby and colleagues (2008) did a study that demonstrated a poor agreement in test results from two WADA-accredited laboratories. Lab A determined recombinant human EPO in all eight subjects, whereas Lab B found no misuse (one sample was negative and seven samples were suspicious).

Conclusion

The Caribbean has little or no input in the development of the various anti-doping tests; therefore, doping tests are developed that might not correct for biochemical variations in Caribbean athletes. It is, therefore, imperative to have a biological profile of elite athletes that can possibly explain some variants that might be unique to particular athletes. Biochemical indices outside of the normal range can be due to physiological or pathological conditions (WADA 2008). However, after a doping offence is implied, it is difficult to repair an athlete's reputation. Based on the performance of the Jamaicans at the recent Beijing Olympics and the World Championships in Berlin, it is imperative that haematologic profiling of our athletes be done. We must be able to protect the athlete's credibility based on sound scientific data if we are reasonably certain that a doping offence has not been committed.

References

Agrawal, A. 1997. Gendered bodies: The case of the "third gender" in India. *Contributions to Indian Sociology* 31 (2): 273–97.

Dehennin, L. 1994. The origin of physiologically high ratios of urinary testosterone. *Journal of Endocrinology* 1 (42): 353–60.

Frazer, C., and E. Harris. 1989. Generation and application of data on biological variation in clinical chemistry. Critical Review of Clinical Laboratory Science 27 (5): 409–37.

Johnson, C. 2004. Clinical practice guidelines for chronic kidney disease in adults: part II: Glomerular filtration rate, proteinuria, and other markers. *American Family Physician* 70:869–76.

Lundby, C., N. Achman-Andersen, J. Thomsen, A. Norgaard and P. Robach. 2008. Testing for recombinant human erythropoietin in urine: Problems associated with current anti-doping testing. *Journal of Applied Physiology* 105:417–19.

Maughan, R. 2005. Contamination of dietary supplements and positive drug tests in sport. *Journal of Sports Sciences* 23 (9): 883–89.

Nakanishi, K. 1974. *Natural products chemistry*. Vol. 1. New York: Academic Press.

Perry, S., T. Byers, R. Yip and S. Margen. 1992. Iron nutrition does not account for the hemoglobin differences between blacks and whites. *Journal of Nutrition* 122 (7): 1417–424.

Purseglove, J.W. 1972. *Tropical crops: Monocotyledons*. London: Longman.

Thirup, P. 2003. Haematocrit: Within subject and seasonal variation. *Sports Medicine* 33 (3): 231–43.

World Anti-Doping Agency. 2008. The World Anti-Doping Code: Models of best practice: Model rules for national anti-doping organizations. V.1.2009 revised code. http://www.wadaama.org/rtecontent/document/code_v2009 _En.pdf.

CHAPTER 16

Intellectual Property and the Business of Sports

KAI-SARAN DAVIS

In August 2008, most of Jamaica and the world were held spellbound, as Jamaican athletes amazed everyone with their immense talent and unforgettable personalities. After walking away from the Beijing Olympics with eleven medals including six gold, our athletes took centre stage in the world and many of the group gained celebrity status overnight.

On the streets of many countries, including Jamaica, a variety of "Usain Bolt" and "Shelly-Anne" T-shirts were available for sale. Moreover, the lightning bolt symbol could be found on shoes, socks and cups. On and after 21 August 2008, the day Usain Bolt ran his final race and held up his characteristic lightning Bolt sign for the last time in Beijing, the Jamaica Intellectual Property Office received a number of applications for registration of trademarks from around the world. These applications were for products very conveniently making reference to lightning bolts, the name "Usain" and the term "To di Worl".

During the Olympic excitement and in its immediate aftermath, many older and former athletes bemoaned the fact that in the past, after major sporting events, their pictures were often freely reproduced in widely circulated print media by companies seeking to benefit commercially without their (the athletes') permission or, even worse, without their knowledge. Many of these former athletes were at pains to point out that while businesses benefited from their images, names and personalities, these athletes were often close to penniless.

Sports: A Business

Although the English dictionary describes sport as "physical activity and/or skill that is governed by a set of rules or customs and often engaged in competitively", the modern media has made us more than aware that sport is also a multimillion-dollar business. The players in this business are not just the athletes but the attorneys-at-law, sports agents, television stations, other media and sports clubs. In addition to this, there are hundreds of professions and trades that obtain indirect financial benefits from sports. It is therefore unfortunate that, too often, especially in our country, athletes' commercial worth is not fully understood. Lest we forget, without these key players there is no game.

So how do athletes protect their interests in the business of sports? One of the major means of doing so is by ensuring that they protect any creation of their mind that may result from their existence as athletes and personality figures. Also of equal importance is that they must ensure the protection of their image.

Protecting Their Intellectual Property

Athletes should firstly set about the task of ensuring that that which most immediately identifies them is legally protected. The athlete's name can, therefore, be protected by the process of registering it as a trademark. In addition, any other names that are known to identify them in their capacity as a famous or well-known personality should also be protected. This process is a simple one and involves visiting the Jamaica Intellectual Property Office for the purposes of filling out the application and paying the necessary fee. If the mark is accepted for registration, then it will be advertised in the *Jamaica Gazette* or any other appropriate publication that the registrar of industrial property deems fit. This advertising is for the purpose of alerting the Jamaican public that the mark is exclusively that of the registrant (personality). The personality who has carried out this process will also receive a certificate as evidence that the mark is now exclusively their property. Only the owner of the mark will have the right to assign the mark or give a licence to a third party for the mark to be used.

It is also important for sports personalities to be aware that any other creation of their mind may also be considered valuable due to their association with it. These personalities should, therefore, also note that they can register an industrial design for products they may wish to market as well.

An industrial design is the ornamental or aesthetic aspect of an article. The design may consist of three-dimensional features, such as the shape or surface of an article, or of two-dimensional features, such as patterns, lines or colours. An industrial design is often registered so as to ensure that the packaging of a product remains unique and "one-of-a-kind". An example of an industrial design is the Coca-Cola bottle. Depending on what business ventures athletes or celebrities seek to engage in, they might deem it necessary to register a design, therefore ensuring the distinctive look of a product they wish to market.

Finally, athletes should also consider that if they become involved in the artistic field (a track and field athlete or footballer becoming a singer, for example) they will need to protect any artistic, literary or musical work they have created by adhering to the informal copyright system in Jamaica and mailing a copy of their work to themselves via registered mail. When the personality receives the mail, they should not open it unless called on to do so for the purpose of providing proof of ownership.

Protecting and Marketing Their Image

Athletes' images include their reputation as good sportsmen and -women and high achievers as well as their personalities and fame outside of the sporting arena. This is important primarily because athletes may decide that they wish to capitalize on their images in order to market items that may either have their names attached to them or that in some way are connected with their personas.

Athletes should also be concerned about widespread unauthorized usage of their likenesses or other indicia of their identities, because, through these reproductions, others may benefit financially from the athletes' persons at their expense. Even beyond this, however, the right to one's own personality is a basic right of natural justice not to be denied to any human being no matter how well known they are.

Although the Jamaican Trade Marks Act of 2001 may, if invoked, offer protection for the name of a celebrity or sports figure, neither this act nor any other Jamaican legislation expressly provides for protection of the image and personality. Any such legal protection afforded to the athlete is provided by reference to the common law, more specifically the *locus classicus*, *Robert Marley Foundation v. Dino Michelle Ltd* (31 *Jamaica Law Report*, 197–209).

This Supreme Court case heard in 1994 before the late Honourable Justice Neville Clarke established what was, at the time, a little-known civil wrong called the "appropriation of personality". It was also one of the only cases ever heard in the common law world that established that a person's right to their name, image and likeness may extend to their assignees after their death. The case established that such a right entitled the personality to commercially exploit their identity. The case also stated that even if the personality did not exercise this right during their lifetime, their assignees were still entitled to the sole use and exploitation of this identity, after the personality's death. The concept of

assignees possessing this exclusive right despite the personalities themselves not using it for commercial exploitation during their lifetimes was a conclusion also reached in the case of another well-known person, Reverend Dr Martin Luther King Jr (*Martin Luther King Jr Center for Social Change Inc. v. American Heritage Products Inc*).

Robert Marley Foundation v. Dino Michelle Ltd

The Robert Marley Foundation (RMF) was and is a company established in Jamaica with the sole right to use, and authorize others to use, the name, personality, likeness, signature, image, photograph and biography of "Bob Marley". They also operated and continue to operate the Bob Marley Museum. They sell T-shirts and other souvenirs with his likeness or name. Dino Michelle Limited (DM Ltd) carried on business as T-shirt manufacturers producing "fun tops", some of which had images of Bob Marley and the words "Bob 1945–1981". DM Ltd did so without the consent or license of RMF. RMF claimed that DM Ltd misled the public into believing that the latter had an association with Bob Marley and also that DM Ltd had appropriated RMF's exclusive right to the Bob Marley image and name.

The court's decision included the fact that when a person has a persona that is commercially marketable, another person should not be allowed to take unauthorized commercial advantage of that persona. This followed closely in line with the principle of unjust enrichment, which dictates that no person should unjustly benefit at the expense of another. The right, therefore, accorded the celebrity a right similar to that of a property right. Also of note is that, as the law recognized rights attached to the goodwill of a business, it also recognized the rights attached to the goodwill generated by the celebrity personality.

In support of his decision, Justice Clark pointed out two important points in the discussion about the right to one's personality:

1. The right of the celebrity must be protected regardless of whether they exploited their celebrity while alive, as it would be wrong to put a premium on exploitation by favouring protection for those who did exploit their personality in life over those who did not. He stated that the person who did not exploit their image, if anything, should be entitled to even more protection after death from those to whom he has not expressly entrusted the care of his image.

2. If a celebrity's name and likeness were to enter the public domain at death, the value of any existing commercial contract while the personality was alive would be severely limited since death is, very often, an unplanned event.

Athletes and their families and personal supporters must be proactive in ensuring that their rights are enforced, and in particular that others do not wrongly profit from their existence. This is not a task that anyone else can champion if the athletes and their loved ones do not make it their business to do so. It is up to every one of us to take a proactive approach in protecting our rights to our images, names and likenesses. If we do not enforce our right to control the very essence of what defines who we are to the world, then no one else can do it for us.

Contributors

Rachael Irving, PhD, is a research fellow in the Department of Basic Medical Sciences, Faculty of Medical Sciences, University of the West Indies, Mona, Jamaica. She is a member of the International Centre for East African Running Science (ICEARS), and the American College of Sports Medicine.

Vilma Charlton, OD, BSc, MSc, is a lecturer at the Institute of Education, University of the West Indies, Mona, Jamaica. She is a physical education specialist, an Olympian, president of the Olympians Association of Jamaica, third vice-president of the Jamaica Amateur Athletic Association and a member of the American Association of Physical Education, Recreation, Sport and Dance.

Helen Asemota, PhD, is a professor of biochemistry, University of the West Indies, Mona, Jamaica. She also serves as professor and head of the Nanotechnology Department, Shaw University, North Carolina, United States.

Jimmy Carnegie, BA, MSc, was a retired principal of Jamaica College and former principal of G.C. Foster College. He was an avid historian, author, sport commentator and jazz enthusiast.

Patrick Cooper, BA, was a journalist and businessman. He served in 1968 as part of the speech-writing team for the US Democratic vice-presidential candidate Edmund Muskie, and later as speech writer to Michael Manley, former prime minister of Jamaica.

Kai-saran Davis, LLB, is an attorney-at-law and manager of Trade Marks, Industrial Designs and Geographical Indications Directorate at Jamaica Intellectual Property Office (JIPO).

Bobby Fray, LLB, is a sports journalist and has worked with KLAS Sports, Hot 102 and the Jamaica Broadcasting Corporation. He has covered many Olympic Games.

Carron Gordon, MSc (Rehabilitation Science), BSc, PT, is head of Physical Therapy, Department of Basic Medical Sciences, Faculty of Medical Sciences, University of the West Indies, Mona, Jamaica.

Fred Green, BSc (Physical Education), is a retired physical education teacher, former secretary of the Intersecondary Schools Sports Association, past sports director of the University of the West Indies and officials' instructor for the International Association of Athletics Federations. He has been associated with Boys' and Girls' Championships for more than fifty years.

Aggrey Benjamin Irons, MBBS, DPM, MD, is a psychiatrist and former senior medical officer at Bellevue Hospital in Kingston, Jamaica.

Donovan McGrowder, PhD, MSc, is senior lecturer, Department of Pathology, Faculty of Medical Sciences, University of the West Indies, Mona, Jamaica, and consultant in chemical pathology at the University Hospital of the West Indies.

Errol Morrison, OJ, MD, PhD, FRCP (UK), FACP, FRSM (UK), FRSH, is president of the University of Technology, Jamaica, and former pro-vice chancellor and dean of the School of Graduate Studies and Research at the University of the West Indies, Mona, Jamaica. He is also an endocrinologist.

Gail Nelson, MPhysio (Cardiothoracic), DipPT, is lecturer in physical therapy, Department of Basic Medical Sciences, University of the West Indies, Mona, Jamaica.

Yannis Pitsiladis, BA (Hons), MMedSci, PhD, FACSM, is a reader in exercise physiology at the University of Glas-gow and director of the International Centre for East African Running Science (ICEARS).

Sharmella Roopchand-Martin, DPT, MSc (Rehabilitation Science), BSc, PT, is a lecturer in physical therapy, Department of Basic Medical Sciences, University of the West Indies, Mona, Jamaica.

Robert A. Scott, PhD, is a career development fellow, Medical Research Council Epidemiology Unit, Cambridge University.

Marilyn
MONROE

To
JoJo
William

Tom ex

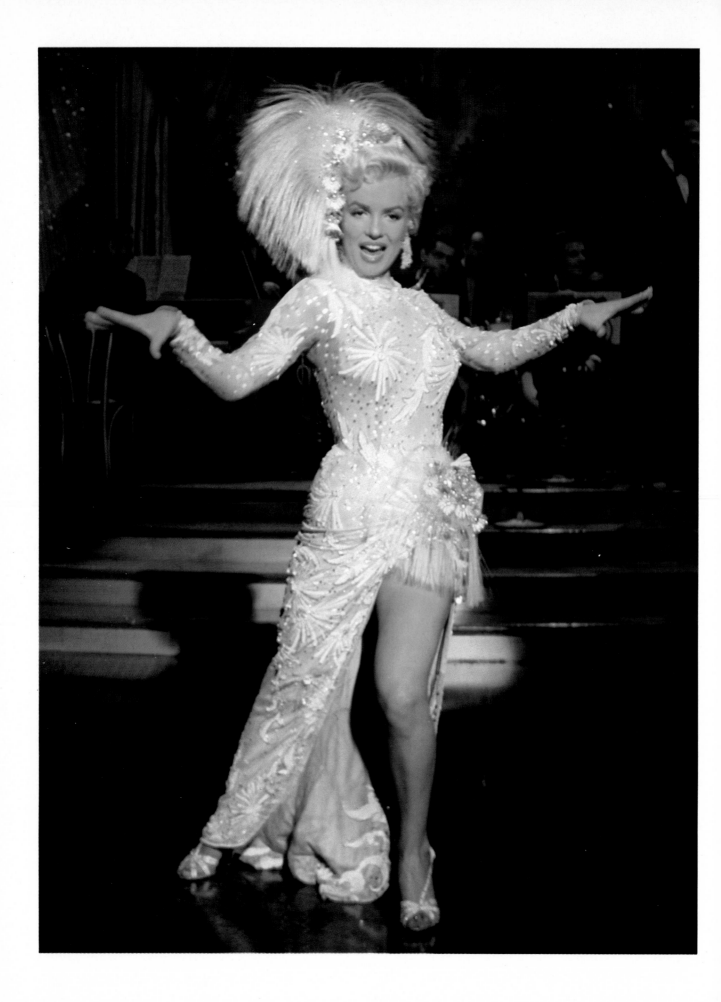

Marilyn MONROE

TOM HUTCHINSON

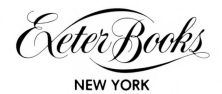

Exeter Books

NEW YORK

Photographic acknowledgments

All photographs published in this book are from the Kobal Collection, London, with the exception of the following: Camera Press, London 66 top, 66 below, 67; Central Press, London 7, 42; Colour Library International, London 59, 75; Popperfoto, London 9 top, 43, 52, 64, 68, 78; Rex Features 6, 8, 12, 19, 21, 25, 34, 44, 49, 50, 61 top, 73, 74 below, 77.

Front cover: Kobal Collection.
Back cover: *Gentlemen Prefer Blondes* (Twentieth Century-Fox). Kobal Collection.
Frontispiece: *There's No Business like Show Business* (Twentieth Century-Fox). Kobal Collection.

CONTENTS

NORMA JEAN

The uncomplicated glamour of one of the screen's last and most potent love goddesses, Marilyn Monroe.

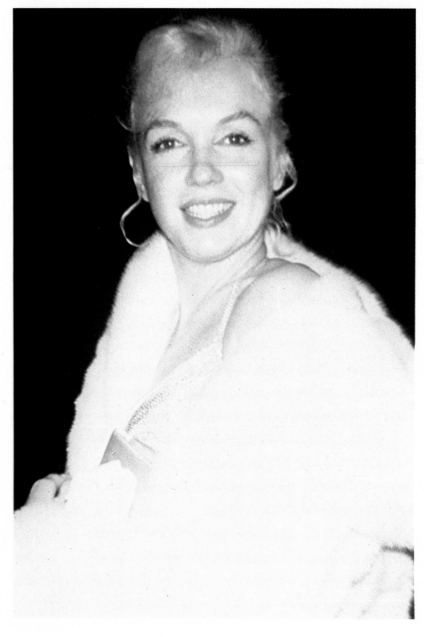

She was the girl who had everything – and nothing. She had all to live for, yet her death was called 'probable suicide'. She, who could have had her pick of any man in the world, died alone on a Saturday night – the night when everyone had a date. Everyone that is apart from her.

All her life Marilyn Monroe was a paradox, a contradiction in the terms that Hollywood set her. She was the most famous sex symbol in the world, a blonde bombshell detonating in all men's dreams as an implication of attainable femininity. Yet there was an interior innocence about her which, like a watermark, gleamed through that surface gloss of glamour.

She came on with the presence of royalty. When I first saw her she had arrived in London to make *The Prince and the Showgirl* with Laurence Olivier, and they sat on a dais at the end of the hotel's banqueting room inviting questions from the assembled Pressmen, for all the world as though the two of them were Government officials or statesmen. Other stars would hold receptions at which they mingled with journalists, but Olivier and Monroe were just that bit above that sort of thing. It was not so much condescension, as the natural order of things.

During the filming of *The Prince and the Showgirl* I met her a couple of times, in more intimate circumstances, at the house she had rented just outside London. There were always 'courtiers' around, of course; often, she said, she relied on them to make her decisions for her. Often they would answer for her, and she would look blankly on, like a ventriloquist's beautiful doll that has forgotten its lines.

Looking back at her too-short life, it does seem that too rarely did she write her own lines: she always appeared dependent upon others. Yet in her movies how different a character, how self-sufficient and, even, self-mocking, she could be, with those pouting lips and that bottom-wiggle.

By her movies shall we know her: that style, that languorous, aware personality, that sense of wit. Even in films that might be termed disaster areas, she was always a saving grace, by very virtue of being in them in the first place. We felt her vulnerability as though it were a physical atmosphere; instinctively we were always on her side. In *The Asphalt Jungle* she plays the young mistress of the much older Louis Calhern, who is involved with a robbery. 'Some sweet kid'

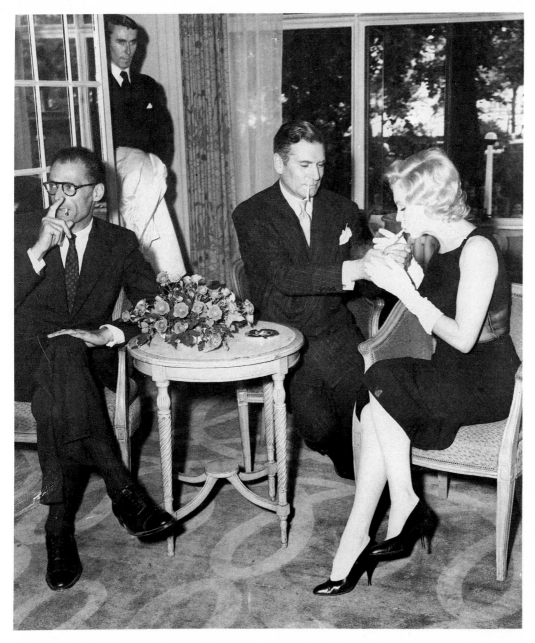

Marilyn Monroe at a press conference at the Savoy Hotel, London, in 1956, when she came to England to make *The Prince and the Showgirl.* Lighting a cigarette for her is her co-star, perhaps the world's greatest actor, Sir Laurence Olivier, and to the left is her husband, one of the world's leading playwrights, Arthur Miller.

is his comment on her, meant without sarcasm. It was always how we thought of her.

The end of a life usually means the end of a career, the celebrity lingering on in the minds and rituals only of the faithful adherents, as in the cases of Elvis Presley and James Dean. Paradoxically, it seems that Marilyn's aftermath has added fresh impetus to the interest in her. Biographies have been written either as straightforward accounts or, most notoriously in the case of Norman Mailer, as *faction.* Films have been made around her life with look-alike Marilyns. The public interest in her is still at peak point. Why should this be so?

It is given to some rare ones to become myths while they are still alive, but Marilyn has become a legend after her death. This may be because we sense in her that inno-

cence I spoke of, that quality of allure combined with an unknowing sensuality. She gave her films a sense of occasion that still survives no matter how many times we see them on television or up there on the bigger screen. Our continuing interest is because we sense in her some of the contradictions within ourselves: the difference between what we think we are and what others see.

Marilyn's life and career spelt out that difference between the image and the imaginer. She has been called one of the last great romantic figures of the screen, but we know that behind that romantic ideal was a woman who was far different from that outward conception. That, unconsciously, we understand and sympathize with. Marilyn Monroe was all things to men and to women. Yet she was just the one thing with which they could all identify. That is her paradox. That is why her legend is indestructible.

On 1 June 1926 the talk at Consolidated Film Industries in Hollywood was about the absence of Gladys Mortensen. Gladys was a section head in the firm, which spliced film together for the principal studios; she was as liked as any other boss would be, but perhaps there was a touch of malice to spike the gossip with a sense of how are the mighty fallen. For Gladys was not at work because she was having a baby and she wasn't married to the man who was reputed to be the father: one of the firm's junior executives.

Gladys had been married once and already had two children, who were living with relatives, but she was now single and fancy-free. That fancy, though, was now no longer as free, but was tethered to a hospital bed as she gave birth to a little girl, Norma Jean,

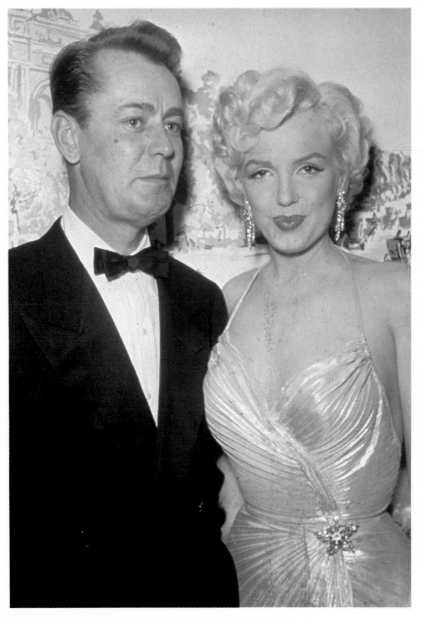

The Hollywood film-cutter's daughter who became a legend with the superstar of an earlier generation, Alan Ladd.

the girl who was to become Marilyn Monroe. Marilyn herself never liked the name of Norma: 'I think I was christened it because Norma was a very box-office name around that time, what with Norma Shearer, that sort of thing. But it sounded too Normal, if you know what I mean.'

The name, though, was typical of Gladys's addiction to the movies; she was star-struck in the most infatuated of ways. She would have liked to have been on screen herself, but Consolidated Film Industries was the nearest she got to that ambition. There was a time when Marilyn – as she later told 'The King' himself – believed that Clark Gable was her real father. That was something that Gladys had hinted at, perhaps hoping that the wish was father to the need . . .

Norma Jean was a normal, rather podgy baby whose first experience of maternal love was to find herself farmed out to some friends of her mother, the Bolenders, in Hawthorne in the suburb of Los Angeles. Her mother had to return to work, but would visit Norma Jean 'every Saturday'.

That unsettled childhood pattern of being fostered out was to be repeated over and over again throughout her childhood. 'I never had real family', she later recalled, 'although my mother did try her best.' Certainly Gladys was regular with her payments – 25 dollars a month – for Norma Jean's upkeep, and her Saturday visits were welcomed eagerly by the little girl. The visits of her grandmother, Della, had also been looked forward to. But suddenly they stopped. The reason was that Della had been committed to a State Mental Institution, a fact which caused Gladys much disquiet about her own mental condition.

Della's incarceration came about after a period when she was much given to losing her temper and throwing things. Once, she was said to have tried to kill Norma Jean, who was just over 18 months old. She had asked the Bolenders if she could look after the baby for an afternoon. Marilyn later recalled: 'I remember waking up from my nap fighting for my life. Something was pressed against my face. It could have been a pillow. I fought with all my strength.' It seems that Della suddenly became aware of what she was doing and stopped trying to suffocate the child. Marilyn was never to forget it.

It seems that from the moment of her mother's institutionalization, Gladys's depressions, which were already quite profound, got worse. Her father had similarly been confined in a mental hospital and her brother, Marion, had also been stricken with the same illness. She herself felt 'marked out', as she put it.

Then, in 1933, she felt able to bring Norma Jean to live with her in her North

Hollywood home, a large part of which she had rented out to an English couple who worked in and out of films. There Norma Jean learned a wholly different way of life from that of the religious Bolenders, for the talk now was of the gossip of the studios: who was dating whom among the stars, who was up for which role in which movie. The showbiz trade paper, *Variety*, was the new bible which Norma Jean learned to accept with as much enjoyment as the former real Bible which the Bolenders had in their front room.

Norma Jean did all the things which little girls at her age did, and the Great Depression certainly did not concern her overmuch. She noticed that the corners were occupied by people lounging around, looking for something to do; it certainly never occurred to her that they were out of work. Then one day calamity struck her in a way that, ever after, she was to maintain, made her 'a natural victim'. Her mother Gladys was committed to a mental hospital. Her hysterias had been getting worse; the neighbours had complained: strait-jacketed and raving she was taken away. When Marilyn came home from school she was told: 'Your mother's gone away for a time.' In recent months Gladys had been working as a film cutter for Columbia Studios and for some weeks the Studios kept on paying her salary. But that dried up eventually. Late in 1935, Norma Jean was admitted to the Los Angeles Orphan Home Society.

She remembered her nearly two years there with some bitterness, but in fact it appears that conditions were not deliberately cruel or brutal; it was just that, being a large establishment, there was little time for individual attention and love. The directress of the home was reported later to have said that 'with some girls our orphanage worked and they were happy in it. But Norma Jean was not that sort of child.' However it was there that she learned how to apply make-up, which was kindly provided by the staff, and how to day-dream: an escape hatch from a reality which she resented very deeply. Occasionally, she asked how her mother was and was told a complacent 'fine'. But in truth, she was now virtually to be separated completely from Gladys. In later years she would rarely discuss her mother, perhaps feeling the same sense of betrayal that Charles Dickens felt when his mother put him to the blacking factory when he was young: he never discussed that painful time of his life and his only reference to it was sour and rancid as though the memory still rankled.

Part of Norma Jean's day-dreaming was of the movies, of course, because the or-

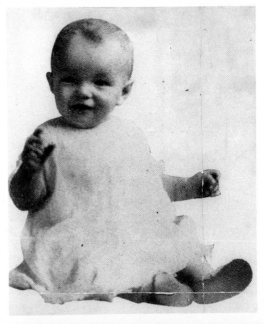

Two pictures of the young Norma Jean. On the left (reproduced from a newspaper photograph), the baby, and below, a happy portrait of the five-year-old Norma Jean taken in 1931, when she was living with her foster parents, the Bolenders.

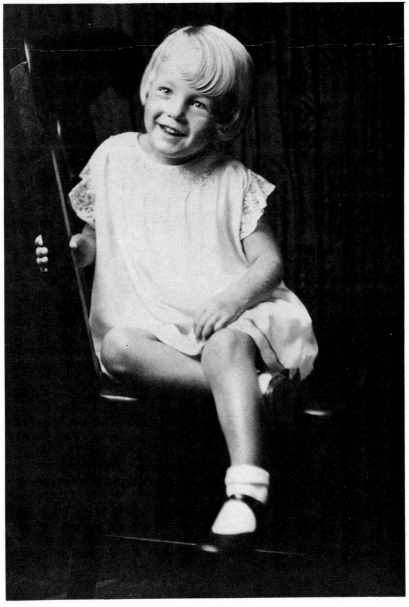

phanage girls were allowed to visit the cinema. She resented being called an 'orphan' because her mother was still alive, but she did not resent the cinema: that was a further exit for her from immediate reality.

Eventually came release. Grace McKee, an old friend of her mother at Columbia Studios, was appointed guardian of Norma Jean, and she went to live with Grace and her husband, Doc Goddard. She was asked if she wanted to take on the new name of her adoptive family, but never got round to doing so. In the Goddard family there was, for Norma Jean, some of the stability that had been so absent from most of her life. But, even under such secure wraps of family life, the rain came in.

Doc Goddard was a man who liked his liquor and was quite often inebriated. Norma Jean was fond of him, but aware that he could not be trusted entirely. Sure enough, one day he made what she considered to be a pass at her. There was a violent scene. Certainly, in later years, Marilyn dramatized it into a near-sexual assault and other writers have wondered just how far the pass had gone. That she was on friendly terms with him afterwards – just never letting herself be left alone with him – shows that it cannot have been the completely physical attack that she sometimes talked about.

Goddard's attention may very well have been attracted by Norma Jean at around this time, for she had burgeoned into a delightful and attractive adolescent girl. She was cute in a dimpled sort of way and she was only too well aware that her figure was of the kind that men and boys turned round to whistle at in the streets. War had broken out with Germany and Japan and pin-ups of Betty Grable and Alice Faye were the tops with servicemen; Marilyn has been reported as saying: 'I strove to look like Betty Grable, but I thought that Alice Faye had more class to her looks.'

The family were now living in West Los Angeles, with Grace's mother, Ana, and things seemed to be moving along as happily for Norma Jean as for other girls of pubescent age at that time. Events, though, now moved precipitately forward, occasioned by the fact that Doc Goddard had the offer of promotion and a job elsewhere. Other writers have said that Grace planned what was to happen now with cool deliberation, because she realized that Norma Jean would be a hindrance in the move to Goddard's new place of employment. Whether she did or not, the event was to mark Norma Jean's progress into a new aspect of life. And it concerned the old movie cliché – the boy next door.

Actually, Jim Dougherty lived a few doors away but he and Marilyn knew each other as neighbours. When Grace asked him 'as a favour' to double-date with Norma Jean for a local dance he agreed casually enough. Jim was very much the outdoor type, enjoyed all things to do with the fresh air. Norma Jean was happy enough to go along with that as their relationship developed. For it *was* developing. Came the time when Grace suggested to the elder Doughertys that the two of them were such an 'item' that they might as well get married.

Somehow or other, that was what was projected. Was it part of a deep-laid plot on Grace's behalf? Marilyn thought so when talking about it later. Whatever the truth, the fact is that on 18 June 1942 the marriage took place. The Goddards, who were by now in Virginia, were unable to come, but the Bolenders turned up. Norma Jean's mother, though, was absent, having been moved to a new mental home.

It is worth noting the ages of the bride and groom. He was 18 and Norma Jean was only just 16. Somebody remarked: 'Are they old enough to know what they are doing?' and somebody else answered: 'Well, it's wartime.' That was the all-purpose excuse.

Jim Dougherty was working at the Lockheed plant as an engineer, and the pressure was so great on production demands that there was no time for a honeymoon. Instead the newly-weds went weekend-fishing at Sherwood Lake near where they lived in Sherwood Oaks. They must have seemed a very ordinary couple, apparently very much in love, so that when Jim was put on night-shift at Lockheed, she would put a love-note in his lunch-basket so that the night would pass more quickly for him. But Jim had married a girl of sixteen, with a girl's looks and attractions of that age. As their marriage continued he became more and more aware that his wife was growing into quite a beauty: the envy in other men's eyes, when the two of them went to dances or, even, walked down the street was becoming oppressive.

That this niggled at him he was afterwards readily to admit. He had the feeling that others were to feel later: that Marilyn – Norma Jean as she was then – belonged to other people besides himself. And, in belonging to all she really belonged to none. But Norma Jean, certainly at that time, thought that their love could stand the invasion of other men's attentions, especially when those attentions were confined to frank glances of admiration for the way her body had developed. That relationship, though, was now going to be put to the test. And it was a test that it could not withstand.

10

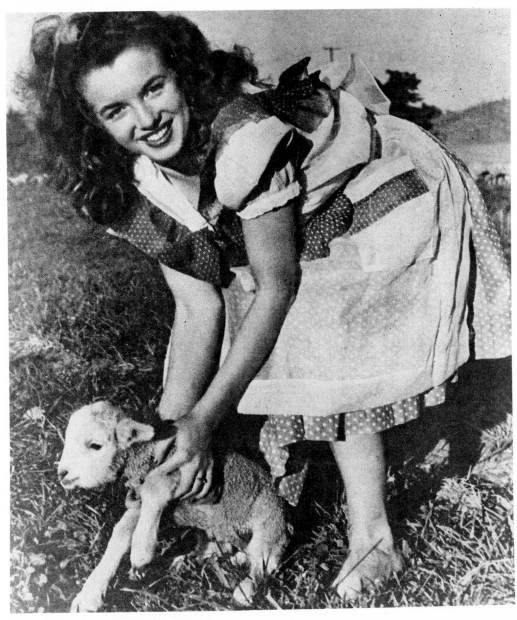

Norma Jean in 1945, when she was 19 years old. Although she looks so young, she had been married for three years, was about to obtain a divorce and was already launched on a modelling career.

Jim Dougherty, feeling more and more conspicuous out of uniform, had joined the Merchant Navy as a physical training instructor, and, eventually, he was shipped out to Australia, later to Italy. The war had taken him away from Norma Jean's proximity. He left her behind with a collie dog, which she adored with the same lavish attention that she had bestowed on a mongrel which she had adopted but which had been shot by a neighbour when she was small. She moved in with Jim's mother and settled back to await the end of the war and her reunification with Jim.

But her mood, without Jim, was restless. She wanted something to do, perhaps even in a patriotic way to feel that she was part of the war effort of which Jim was in the front-line. So she got a job as a parachute-packer. It was simple enough work, but Norma Jean brought such enthusiasm to it that she was graded by her employers as 'excellent'; it was not a grading which was all that much appreciated by the other girls on the factory floor who considered that Norma Jean – who was not all that talkative at lunch-breaks – was just that bit pushy, a bit above herself. Then something else happened which moved Norma Jean further above herself than usual. An army photographer happened.

It was an incident that has been thoroughly documented since. The photographer was David Conover and he was on an assignment at the factory to photograph working girls for *Yank* magazine. There was to be a plurality of females, but Conover's expert eye rested upon Norma Jean – and stayed there. His camera, over the next few days of photography, was exclusively upon her. He was the first to realize just how natural the girl who would become Marilyn Monroe was before a camera: it was the beginning of a love affair with a lens that was to last all her life. Even the director Billy Wilder, who could be very critical of her working methods, said: 'She is one of those stars who bloom into beautiful life when she is in front of the camera. They have this mutual attraction, a mutual admiration society, which we, the audience, witness with gratitude.'

Another photographer saw those photographs that Conover took and, too, was impressed by her naturalness. He asked her if he could photograph her outdoors over a weekend. Norma Jean readily agreed. It was fun being so much the centre of the camera's attention.

Those outdoor photographs came to the attention of Emmeline Snively, who was then the boss of the Blue Book Model Agency. She asked Norma Jean to call and Norma Jean went. Would she like to work a week as a hostess for a steel firm at an Industrial Show? She would indeed. She took time off from the factory, without explaining why, and took over a stand at the show. It was in its way a minor triumph; never had a steel company had so many enquiries. The men flocked with their questions, happily satisfied with the answers supplied to them by this attractive young model.

That was the start of model work, which took off completely after the colour-spread in *Yank* magazine. For a time Norma Jean tried to combine modelling with her job

The sort of picture that was earning Norma Jean a growing reputation among the agencies as a magazine cover girl before she achieved her dream of being in films.

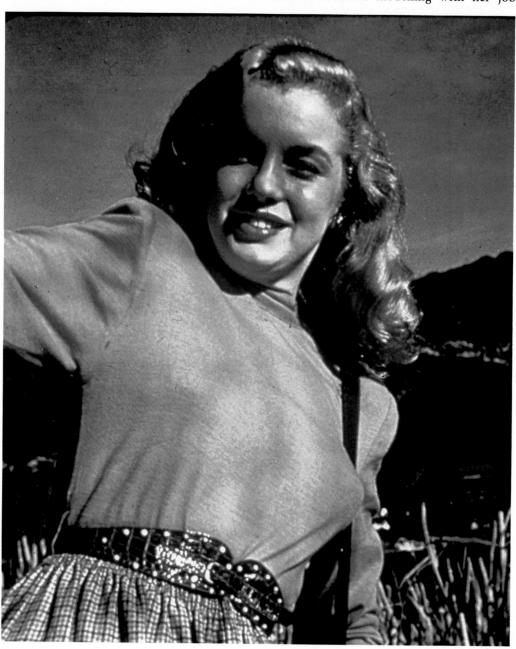

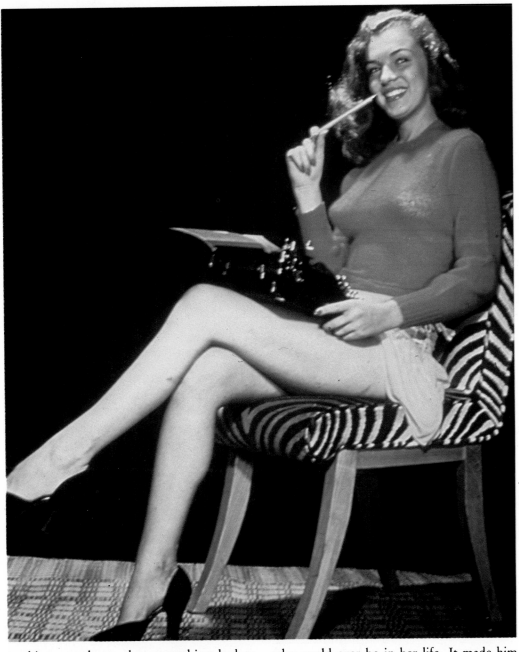

Any excuse was good enough for another stunning picture of the young Marilyn's curves. This unlikely shot of every boss's dream stenographer was taken in 1947, after she had been offered a contract by Twentieth Century-Fox.

packing parachutes, but something had to give and it was parachutes that were sent packing. It was as though Norma Jean had spent all her life waiting for the way her ambition could be defined. Now she knew in which direction her life would be moving. The elder Doughertys were not happy with the situation, so Norma Jean moved out. Her letters to Jim overseas were full of love, but even at that distance he must have felt some sort of disturbance about what was happening, because his mother had written that Norma Jean wasn't 'around all that much'.

When he came home on leave, though, all seemed to be well. He was aware that modelling had its dangers in the contacts with other men, but Norma Jean made it seem and sound as though he were the only man who could ever be in her life. It made him feel more secure. The war was over but Jim was still circling the world on his freighter; he had two photographs of Norma Jean at the side of his bunk: they made her seem nearer.

It was, and perhaps he knew it in his heart of hearts, only an illusion. He said afterwards that he was 'half-expecting' what was about to happen. Norma Jean had already discussed her future with Miss Snively and had been told that top models could – if they were good enough – get contracts as actresses with one or other of the major film studios. It was then and there that Norma Jean decided that the broad direction in which her career was now heading could be even further refined to a single track – that leading to stardom.

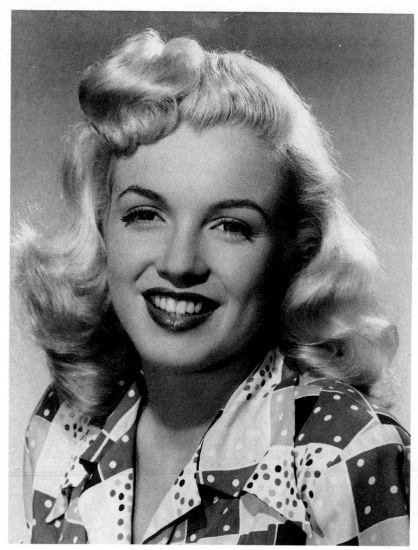

Pictures of her protégée appeared on cover after cover of magazines; she posed for calendars; she learned the trade of knowing just how to look for the camera. She was, in a work-drenched sort of way, very happy.

She even went to studios for auditions, but nothing came of them. Then one day in July 1946 she went for an audition to Ben Lyon, the casting director of Twentieth Century-Fox. Lyon had been a film star himself, then a comedian – with his wife, Bebe Daniels – in Britain during the war. He had an eye for talent. He saw it immediately in Norma Jean. She was given a film test and Lyon recalled that the spark he had felt on meeting her was suddenly up there on the screen, but multiplied a thousandfold. 'She glowed; she was tremendous, although very nervous.' Norma Jean was offered a contract starting at 75 dollars a week. But there was one small point. Her name. It didn't sound right.

Lyon remembered a former entertainer called Marilyn Miller. Marilyn was an interesting name. Norma Jean was asked if she liked it. Only, said Norma Jean, for the last time Norma Jean, if she could couple it with her grandmother's name. Which was? 'Monroe', said Marilyn Monroe.

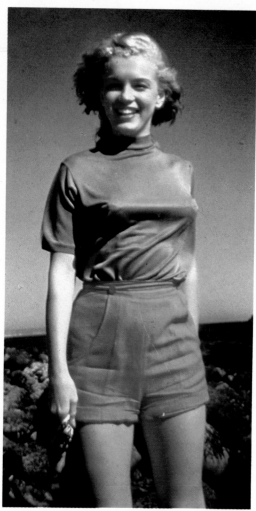

Above: The finished studio image of the young starlet. This photograph of Marilyn was taken after a make-up session at Columbia Studios for *Ladies of the Chorus*.

Right: A glamour shot of the early Monroe, making the most of her figure, taken around 1947–48.

Jim Dougherty received the attorney's letter while his ship was in Shanghai. A divorce was called for. The marriage, which had been quietly expiring, was over.

The reasons may be hard-hearted, but they were complete enough reasons in themselves: studios just did not sign up potential female talent if that talent was married. The reason: the possibility of pregnancy. A starlet, after all, was an investment for the future and business is business – a business which could not afford to let itself be swollen out of success and into bankruptcy by an act of nature which could be forestalled.

So the Doughertys were divorced. Norma Jean was 'orphaning' somebody else for a change. She who had all her life been left by one person or another, who later said that she had felt manipulated during all the early part of her life, was herself leaving another human being. It was a pity, but there it was. 'He was a kind man', she recalled later, 'but, you know, we had nothing in common.'

Meanwhile back at her career, Miss Snively was conscientiously applying herself.

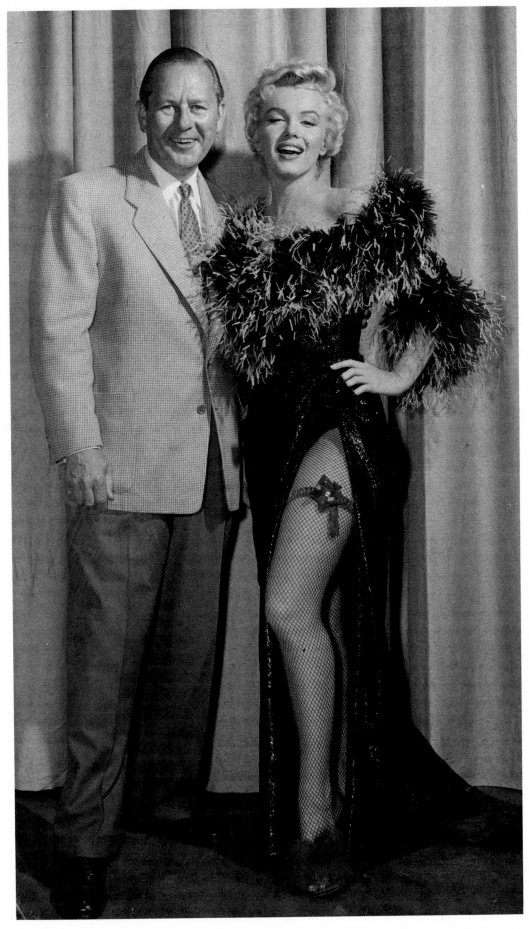

Marilyn in 1955, wearing one of her costumes for *The Seven Year Itch* (Twentieth Century-Fox), with the studio's casting director, Ben Lyon, who had realized her screen potential when giving her a test in 1946.

THE GOOD MR HYDE

A new name? Perhaps Marilyn hoped that, along with it, there would be a new switch of direction to her life: that it would, at last, have some purpose against the feeling that dogged her all this early part of her life – and to some extent to the end of it – that she was either drifting or being manipulated. It was not to be, of course. Marilyn found, like so many other aspiring starlets around this time of 1947, that a film studio was a factory just as the parachute factory was, and everything was geared to the product. She wasn't part of, or involved with, that product yet. She was on the periphery of Fox's real activities.

Of course, as an attractive girl with an undoubtedly real and luminous personality, she made friends . . . usually men friends. Principal among these was Joseph M. Schenck, an executive producer at Fox, who at the age of 69 had a reputation for womanizing and a power which made him a formidable personality among those in the know on the Fox lot. 'He was a cute little guy', Marilyn was reported later to have said

of him, a description with which his enemies would have agreed only so far as the diminutive aspect of his appearance went. Cute, he wasn't – to them. But for Marilyn, who graced his dinner parties, he was a provider of at least some good meals.

Marilyn was finding that times were tough; the crock of gold at the end of the rainbow, that she had expected her contract to be, was buried too deep. Then came what was officially her first film, a role which was so fleeting as to be missed if you blinked. It was as a girl on a boat in a film memorably titled *Scudda Hoo! Scudda Hay!* (it was later changed to *Summer Lightning*), a rural hay-ride piece of nonsense which starred June Haver and such hayseeds as Walter Brennan. Natalie Wood got her name on the credits, but you have to look very hard down the cast list to find Marilyn's name. This movie was so distinctly uncelebrated that years later Marilyn could hardly remember what it was about. Similarly, *The Dangerous Years*, which followed (although it was released

This scene from the first film Marilyn made, *Scudda Hoo! Scudda Hay!* (Twentieth Century-Fox), was later cut from the movie. Marilyn and Colleen Townsend prepare to row away while Robert Carnes watches.

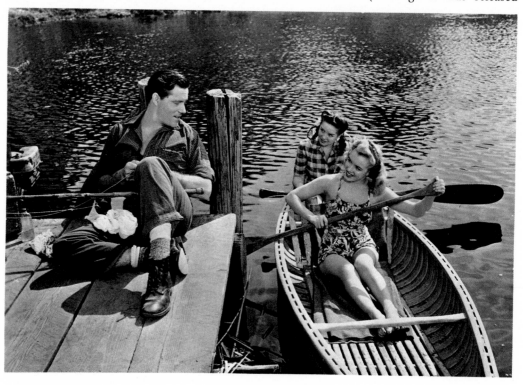

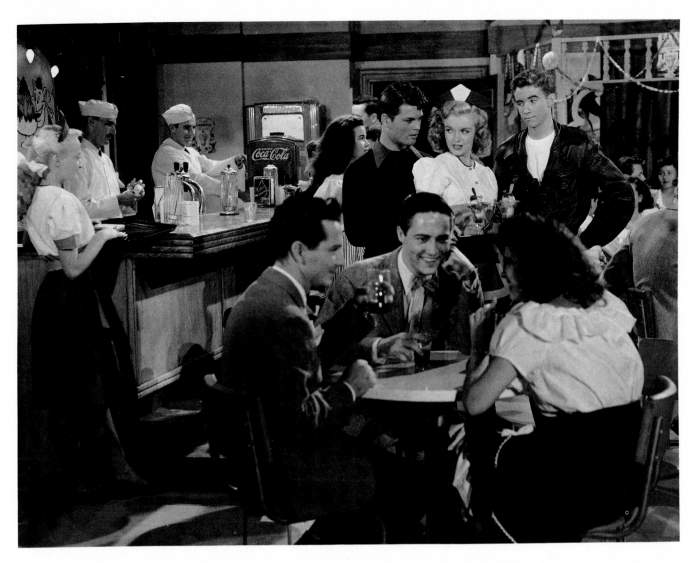

earlier than *Scudda Hoo! Scudda Hay!*), again had Marilyn in a small role – a few minutes longer, admittedly, but short enough – as a waitress serving some juvenile delinquents in a café. Thus she had gone along with two strands of cinema's post-war trends: the yearning for ruralism and the belief that anyone below the age of sixteen was up to no good.

Her own life, though, was conforming to no known direction apart from that which states that starlets must suffer as much as possible, so that when they attain the heights writers will have something to write about to explain that top-of-the-tree neurosis. Despite those Schenck dinners, which came albeit infrequently, she was often having to manage on one hamburger and a helping of cottage cheese a day. And even that diet looked as though it would be ended with the news that Fox were not renewing her contract, despite that friendship with Schenck.

However, he was to do her one last, parting favour before she shrugged off those Fox furs – which had turned out to be coney –

not for the last time, but certainly for what she thought then would be the last time. Schenck phoned his friend Harry Cohn, who was boss at Columbia, and said that Marilyn had something which Columbia might appreciate, especially as there was a musical, *Ladies of the Chorus*, being prepared. This, directed by Phil Karlson, was very much a cheapie about burlesque chorines and their offstage romances, and had such forgettable names as Adele Jergens and Rand Brooks in it. It was, however, to be the first film in which Marilyn's name was to figure somewhere up front.

Marilyn's experience of musicals was limited, in fact, to watching those starring Betty Grable or Alice Faye. She had simply no idea how to project that sexy whisper which was later to be amplified as so much a part of her personality. So Columbia assigned a vocal coach, Fred Karger, to help her. It was to become an emotional experience for them both, but from it came Marilyn's lifelong friendship with Fred's mother, Anne, a woman who was always to be her friend and

Marilyn as a waitress between former child stars Dickie Moore and Scotty Beckett in *Dangerous Years* (Twentieth Century-Fox), her first film to be released, although the second she made.

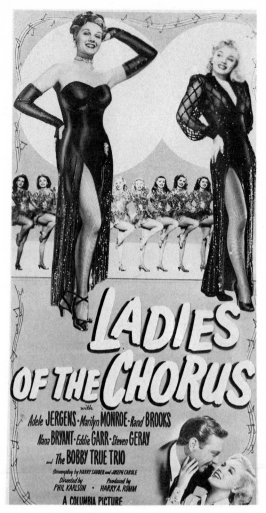

Prominent billing and prominent pictures for Marilyn on a poster for only her third film, *Ladies of the Chorus*, made for Columbia and released in 1949.

always to defend her against any charge of promiscuity. 'She thought of marriage as the natural outcome of mutual passion', she once said.

That it was not to be marriage with Fred was a cause for regret, although work on *Ladies of the Chorus* was so demanding that it drove much of that affair out of her head, as the chores progressed. It was a simple enough story, with Marilyn as the daughter of a burlesque star, who becomes a star of that particular stage in her own right – and then meets and falls for a young society playboy. But even such low-scale rhetoric requires some sort of professional approach. Columbia decided that not only did she require a vocal coach but a dramatic coach as well, Natasha Lytess.

All her life Marilyn was to feel inadequate as an actress, seeking help and guidance from others whom she deemed, rightly or wrongly, to have better knowledge of such things. Natasha Lytess, a grey-haired, dominating woman with a great deal of tough charm, was to be the first of these coaches in Marilyn's career. Miss Lytess admits, in her memoirs, that she took a good deal of interest in her pupils' private lives and tried

to talk Marilyn out of seeing too many men and to persuade her to wear underwear. She was also aware that at her first meeting with Marilyn the girl was 'utterly unsure of herself'. That she was late for the meeting was yet another indication of that lack of belief in herself – or was it, asked Miss Lytess, an example of an ego that would keep others waiting?

Some writers have suggested that, in Natasha Lytess and Anne Karger – as well as many of the others who were to make their way into her life – Marilyn was unconsciously seeking out the mother that she never really had or, at least, who was too remote from her, by way of mental illness, ever to have had any maternal impact. It is a viewpoint that makes more than a case for itself. Throughout her life there were always to be older women, as well as older men, who somehow or other shaped what was to be her destiny.

One of the songs Marilyn sang in *Ladies of the Chorus*, 'Every Baby Needs a Da Da Daddy', might equally well apply to the distaff side of parenthood as well.

Then, in September 1948, came disaster. Columbia dismissed her from the studios. The story, which it must be admitted Marilyn encouraged in later years, was that she had refused the advances of studio boss Harry Cohn, who had exploded into a ferocious display of anger that one of his starlets should thus repudiate him. Cohn's libido was as publicized, and as much a matter of studio concern, as L. B. Mayer's at MGM. If the story of Marilyn's rejection of him is true, there might well be good grounds – in Cohn's mind – for the girl being dismissed: if it got around to his fellow film-tycoons it might well be a laughing matter for them which would undermine his power. And power was the real name of the game: not the name of Marilyn Monroe.

Other girls might well be able to overcome such a wrench from an anchorage with little difficulty or, at least, come to terms with the knowledge that that is the way Hollywood is – especially for young girls out for a career. But Marilyn had had too many severances to take it all with that kind of equanimity. Natasha Lytess reported that Marilyn was distraught, even contemplating the aid of a psychiatrist or the Roman Catholic Church.

She was still very friendly with Natasha Lytess, even staying with her and her daughter at this time, but she was very depressed. There was always modelling work, of course, and it was at about this time in the autumn of 1949 that she worked with photographer Tom Kelley for the calendar that was later to add notoriety to her fame: she posed nude for a photograph that was titled

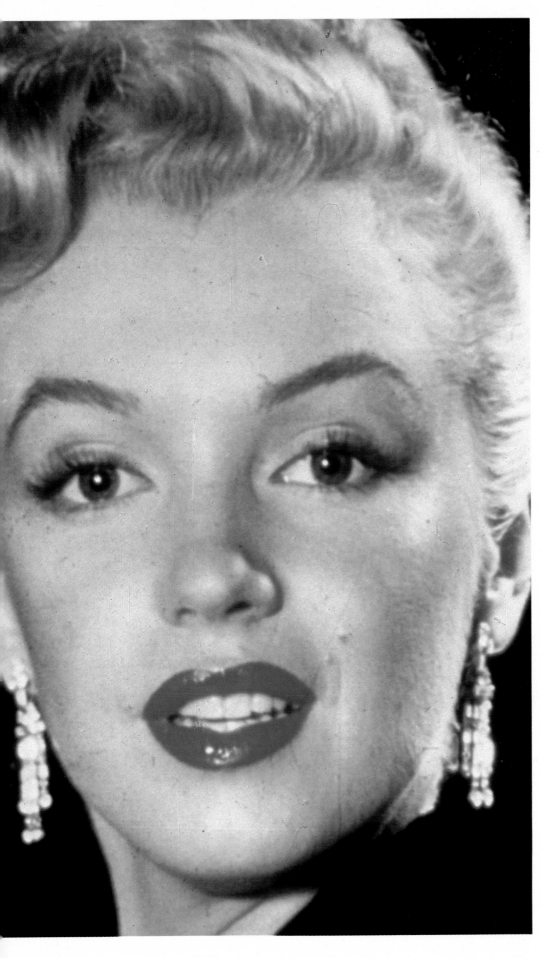

Marilyn in 1950, heavily made up as usual and wearing large drop earrings for her role in *As Young as You Feel* (Twentieth Century-Fox), one of her nine films which were released in 1950 and 1951.

Far right: Marilyn in the first film in which she made a strong impression on the critics. She played the glamorous girlfriend of crooked lawyer Louis Calhern in *The Asphalt Jungle* (MGM), and was sympathetically directed by John Huston.

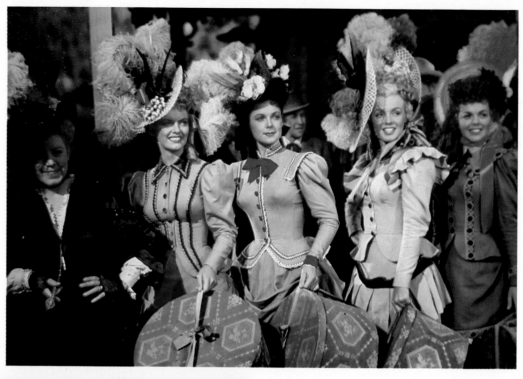

Right: For *A Ticket to Tomahawk* (Twentieth Century-Fox), a light-hearted Western musical, Marilyn (second from right) was one of the chorus line with Joyce MacKenzie, Barbara Smith and Marion Marshall.

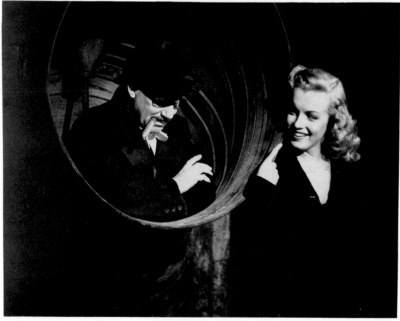

Above: Groucho Marx in *Love Happy* (United Artists) saw the curvaceous Marilyn as the ideal foil for his inimitable brand of lecherous eyebrow-raising.

'Golden Dreams'. But needs must, when the devil of unemployment and the fact of fifty dollars a day from Kelley drives.

Then she slipped back to Twentieth Century-Fox almost unnoticed for a film, starring Dan Dailey, called *A Ticket to Tomahawk*. This was to have been a one-off, but friends spoke up for her and she went into a film called *Love Happy*. It did her no harm around this time to find that she had been mentioned in the syndicated gossip column of Louella Parsons, who wrote kindly about her as a Hollywood orphan who had been brought up within sight of the studios

– and whose ambition it was to go on working there.

Love Happy was an off-the-rails vehicle for the Marx Brothers, a not very bright example of their wonderful absurdity, all about the difficulties – surprise! surprise! – of putting on a musical. Marilyn's role was small enough, to be sure – progressing sexily into Groucho Marx's office and complaining that she was being followed by men, while he leered understandingly at her – but it was to establish her as a presence in the eyes of one man who was to be very important to her at this time. His name was Johnny Hyde and he was a very top-notch agent indeed.

Hyde was a talent scout. And Marilyn, he told everyone, had talent with a capital 'T'. He was also 'love happy' himself.

Johnny Hyde was later said by Marilyn to have been the real reason she became a star. He had a strong belief in her and fought to have her recognized. Marilyn was extremely grateful at the time, and always remained so. What he did was at some sacrifice to himself. Married with four sons – the eldest of whom was about the same age as Marilyn herself – he found his wife filing for divorce and some of his friends believing that he was being taken for a sucker by a scheming, younger woman. He never believed that. As a vice-president of the William Morris Agency, he was an articulate, forceful man of some literacy and discrimination. He realized that Marilyn, like others of his protégées had been, was a woman who had not realized her potential as a person, who lived only for movies. He set out to groom her to be a star,

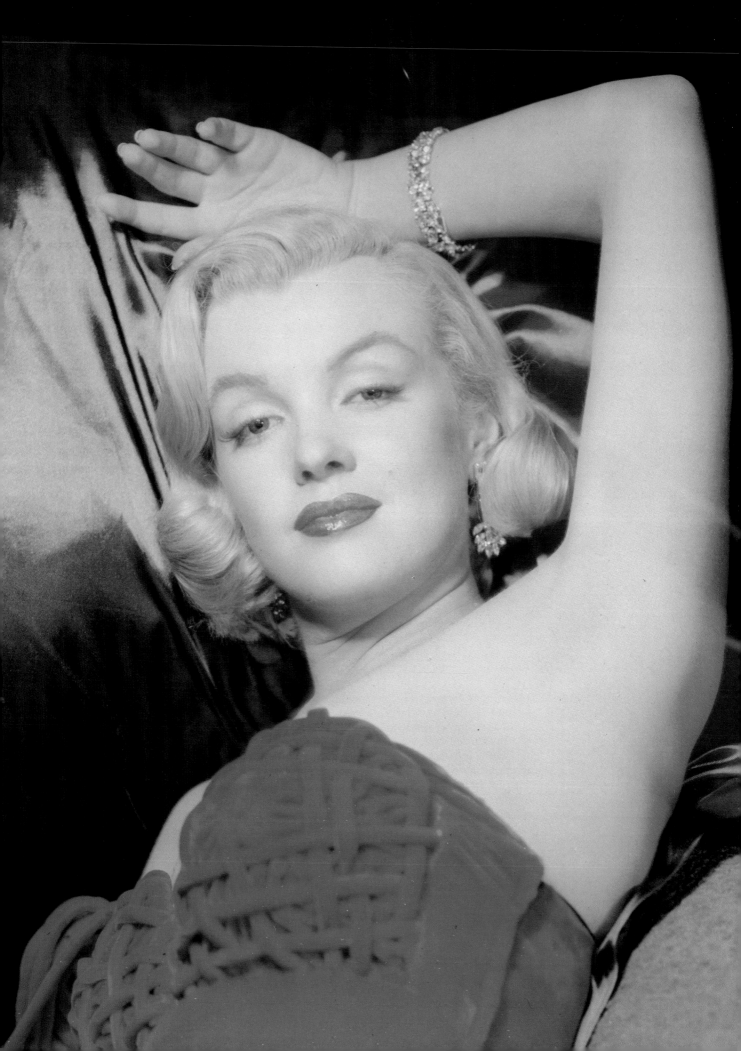

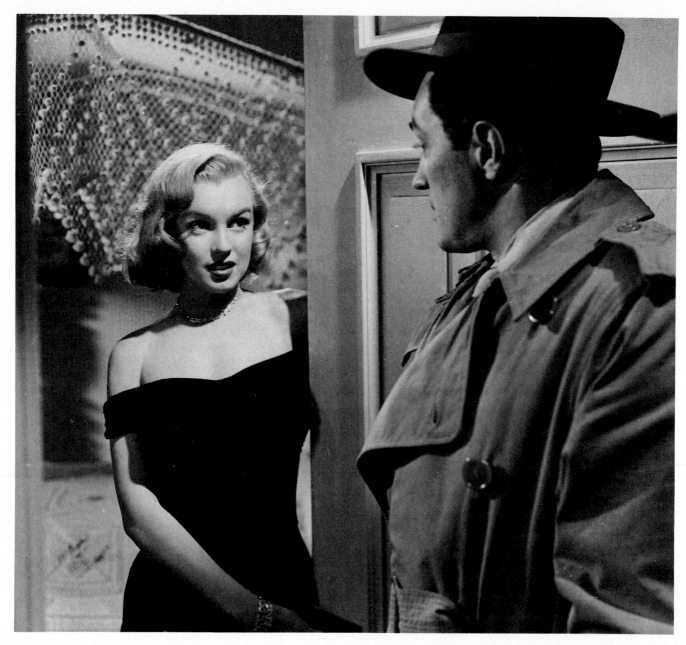

Above: The delectable good-
time girl looking as innocent
as possible in *The Asphalt
Jungle* (MGM).

Right: All cameras, lights and
action as Marilyn, lying on the
couch, plays a close-up scene
with Louis Calhern in MGM's
The Asphalt Jungle.

helping her choose the right dresses and the
correct costume jewellery.

In the film *Marilyn, The Untold Story*,
Johnny Hyde was portrayed by Richard
Basehart, and, certainly, in photographs of
the time, Hyde can be seen to have some of
the looks of the actor. But accounts suggest
his personality did not need to be as forceful
as Basehart's portrayal would have us believe. He was a very wealthy man and had
many friends within the business. One of
these friends was John Huston, the famed
director, who was setting up a movie called
The Asphalt Jungle.

This was a criminal caper movie of an unusual kind for the times in which it was released (1950). It told the story of the robbery
from the point of view of the crooks themselves, characters varying in degrees of

intelligence but always viewed with some
ironic sympathy. Sterling Hayden was the
muscle-man, while Sam Jaffe was the mas-
termind, whose penchant for young girls
leads him to disaster. Involved with them
was the crooked lawyer Louis Calhern who,
with a perpetually ailing wife, has a bubbly
blonde of near-adolescent age as his mistress.
This was the girl to be played by Marilyn in
a movie which endeavoured to show that
crime itself was but a 'left-handed form of
human endeavour'.

Huston recalled that he had wanted to test
Marilyn for his previous movie, *We Were
Strangers*, but 'circumstances kept getting in
the way'. He now tested her for *The Asphalt
Jungle* and decided that her projection of
insecure seductiveness was exactly right for
the role.

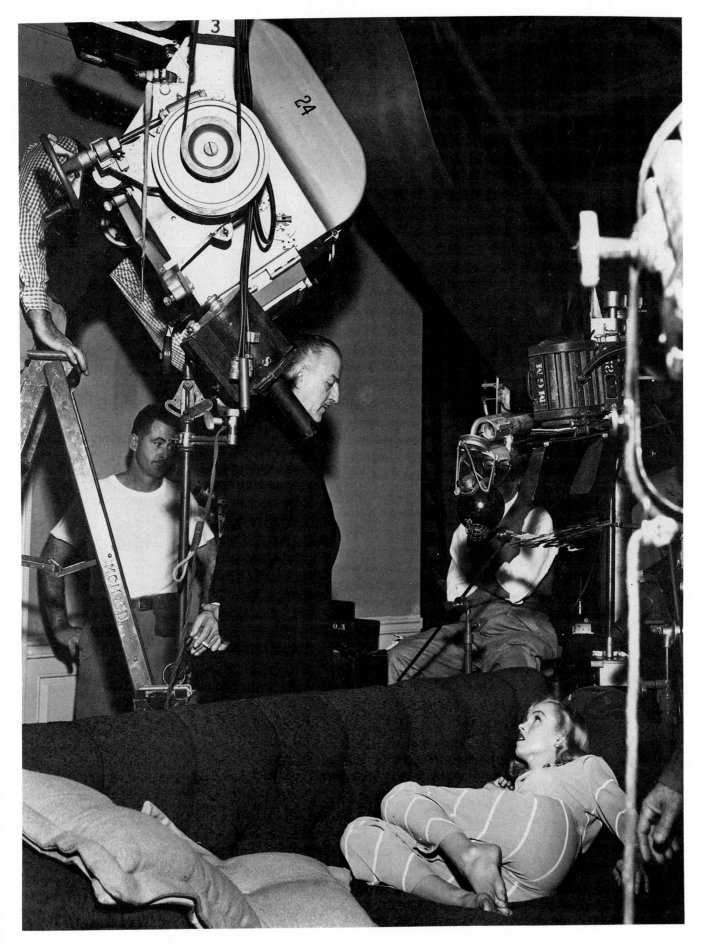

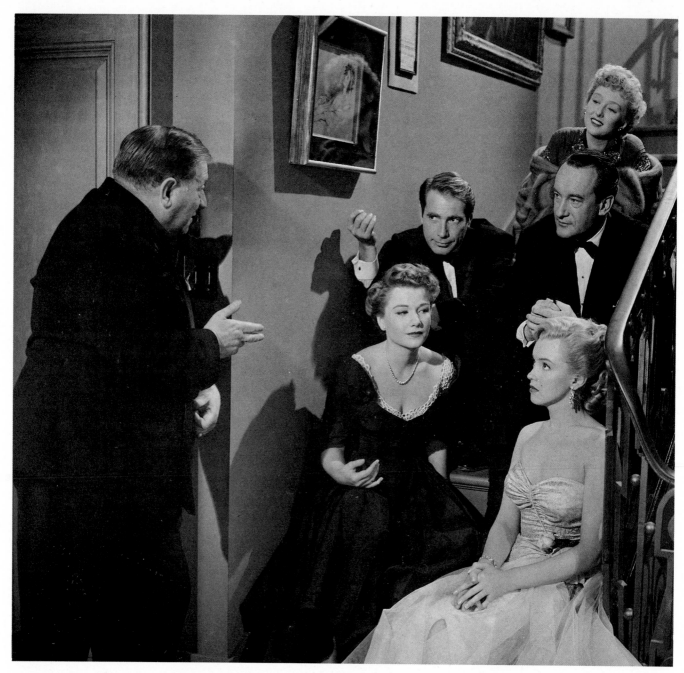

Marilyn played the small part of a guest at a theatrical party in the very successful *All About Eve* (Twentieth Century-Fox), and despite the galaxy of stars was widely noticed by the critics. On the stairs, listening with her to Gregory Ratoff, are Anne Baxter, Gary Merrill, George Sanders and Celeste Holm.

Perhaps he sensed in the part a kind of type-casting for Marilyn, in that she was involved with the distinguished Johnny Hyde, who was himself a much older man with a wife whom he loved. Certainly the performance given by Marilyn suggested more than just the 'bit' parts she had been used to; although small, it nevertheless carried a weight of impact. She was a motivation for the older lawyer to behave in the way he did; she was the girl who, unwittingly, caused him to self-destruct.

There were those, especially at the William Morris Agency, who thought the same motivation could be seen in the relationship between Marilyn and Hyde. He devoted practically all his attention to her, and during

the years 1949–50 she completed around six movies with his help, some of which were negligible in terms of her career but all of which succeeded in helping her image in the public's eye. Perhaps one of the most important of these films was *All About Eve*. This literate and spiky comedy drama of life backstage is about the insecure great actress, played by Bette Davis, who feels her position eventually threatened by the ruthlessly aspiring Anne Baxter, who moves from sycophant to positive rival. At one of those larger-than-life theatrical parties at which people use aphorisms as, in olden times, they might have used rapiers, Marilyn turns up as Miss Caswell, brought by drama critic George Sanders.

Her role was that of a vacuous, on-the-make kind of girl whose overt hankering for a kind of fame was an exact opposite to the covert envy portrayed by Anne Baxter. Marilyn made enough of the part to ensure that critics noticed her, in a film that won general acclaim all around; Bette Davis later recalled that, although Marilyn was on set for only a couple of days, 'she certainly made herself felt. The stills photographers couldn't keep away from her when she was not in front of the movie camera, and she seemed to take great delight in their attentions. No, nobody was jealous of that attention; rather, we were amused. We were all of us, after all, older in the actual business of acting than she was, so we felt she should get the most publicity that she could. Besides, she was so modest when you spoke to her; I rather liked her.'

This was a sympathetic view which was very much opposite to that which the family and friends of Johnny Hyde took of Marilyn. The gossip columnists kept referring to the May-and-December romance, but Hyde would hear nothing against her. He furthered her career with a sacrificial ardour that probably compensated for the physical ardour from which he was severed by a series of heart attacks. He was by now a very sick man. Not so sick, though, that he could not induce Marilyn to have her nose 'bobbed'. That plastic surgery, he thought, was a physical touch which would finally make others appreciate her as much as he did himself. 'Some sweet kid', says Louis Calhern of her in *The Asphalt Jungle*. 'Some sweet kid', Johnny Hyde might well have reiterated in real life.

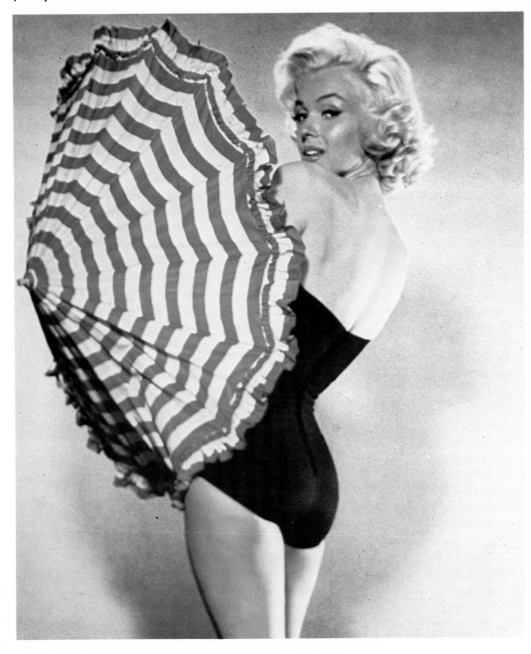

Marilyn's publicity photographs frequently pictured her outdoors on beaches, in bathing suits, wrapped in towels, or, as in this studio shot, making the best of herself with brightly coloured props like a parasol.

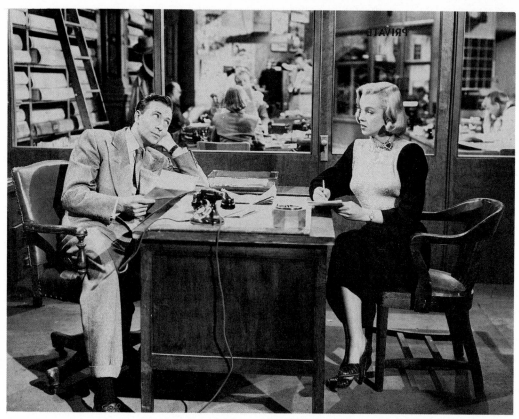

In her early films, Marilyn sometimes provided her own wardrobe, and this outfit, with the carefully arranged clip on the neck, had already been seen in *The Fireball*, when she made *Home Town Story* (MGM), with Jeffrey Lynn.

All this time Marilyn's personality *was* growing in the public consciousness, however; people were aware of her, even if they weren't quite sure about which movie they had seen her in. So big was this appreciation of her that the news that she was being considered for Grushenka in a new visualization of Dostoyevsky's *The Brothers Karamazov* caused interest not only in Hollywood but in the minds of the many men in the street who had so far only seen her as a platinum blonde with a breathy, sexy giggle and a way of walking away from the camera which was a whole scene in itself.

The role of Grushenka eventually went to Maria Schell, which Marilyn afterwards lamented, but Dore Schary of MGM, with whom Hyde had discussed the idea, had been interested – which presupposed that Marilyn was not to be merely simply restricted to mindless, if appealing, blondes. At about this time, November 1951, Johnny Hyde and she finally signed a seven-year contract with Twentieth Century-Fox which would be paying her 750 dollars a week within a year. Darryl F. Zanuck, the boss of Fox, had let it be known that he thought little of Marilyn's potential as a dramatic actress. But obviously he realized she was a product who could be sold, and that, after all, was what film companies were all about. It was as though this act of Johnny Hyde's was rushed through at his request because he realized that soon Marilyn would be once

more on her own, without his protection. That contract would provide a security which, without his being around, she might well need. So, having put her house in order, Johnny Hyde died of a heart attack on 17 December 1951, in Palm Springs.

Natasha Lytess, with whom Marilyn stayed at this time, felt that her charge should not be left alone, so grievously did she seem to be stricken by Hyde's death. Shock seemed to have concussed her with sandbag-force, so that she seemed to have difficulty in hearing questions that were put to her. She was sedated with pills too, pills which were later to become such an important, frightening part of her life. But at least, she said later, they 'helped me to sleep'.

Hyde, seemingly, had asked that Marilyn be treated as one of his family, but that was a request that the family could not tolerate. It was suggested that she would not be welcome at the funeral, but in fact she went along with some friends to say her last farewells. Her sobs were said by members of the family to have been in bad taste, but those who have followed her career might perhaps forgive her for what may well seem a brash mourning to others, for once again she was losing somebody she loved. Moreover, without his guile and charm to protect her, she was very much on her own. Her weeping might just as well have been for herself, and her own vulnerability, as for Johnny Hyde.

THE ROAD AHEAD

Why Marilyn never married Johnny Hyde has never been satisfactorily answered. If she had been a gold-digger impure and simple it would have secured her a fortune from his will; if she were as fond of him as she says that she was at the time then marriage would have consoled his dying days. Perhaps the truth is that at this stage of her life, as she said, 'marriage is such an awful and awesome commitment'. Instead, she was committed to Twentieth Century-Fox. That, too, in its way was 'an awesome commitment'.

Studio head Darryl F. Zanuck has gone on record at this time as insisting that he was not all that enamoured of Marilyn's potential. Indeed, the films that were planned for her were the mixture very much as before: insubstantial and frothy. Her first under the Fox aegis was *As Young as You Feel,* in which she played secretary to Albert Dek-

ker's company president. He has to fire an ageing Monty Woolley who, at 65, is convinced that he can still do something about the company that he helped start. Besides those acting notables, Marilyn was aided by actress Thelma Ritter. That the critics believed that she more than held her own in such august company is indicative of her growing talent for comedy, combined with just a hint of pathos. The film itself is important in any review of Marilyn's life in that this was where she met the man who was to become her third husband: playwright Arthur Miller. He accompanied his friend, the director Elia Kazan, who was really checking up on his former editor, Harmon Jones, who was directing *As Young as You Feel.* In 'The Tragedy of Marilyn Monroe' the writer Fred Lawrence Guiles says that after this meeting with Miller she said: 'It was like running into

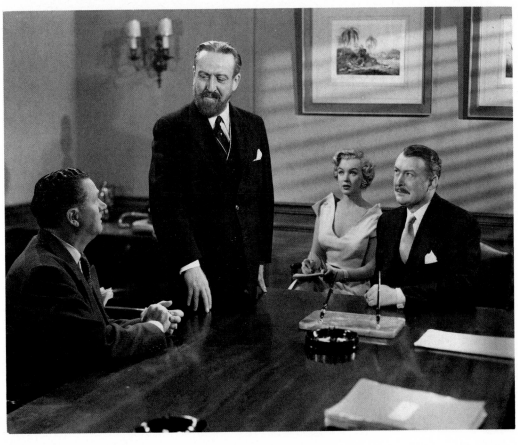

Marilyn in a comedy of the business world, *As Young as You Feel* (Twentieth Century-Fox). With her in this scene are, from the left, Wally Brown, Monty Woolley and Albert Dekker.

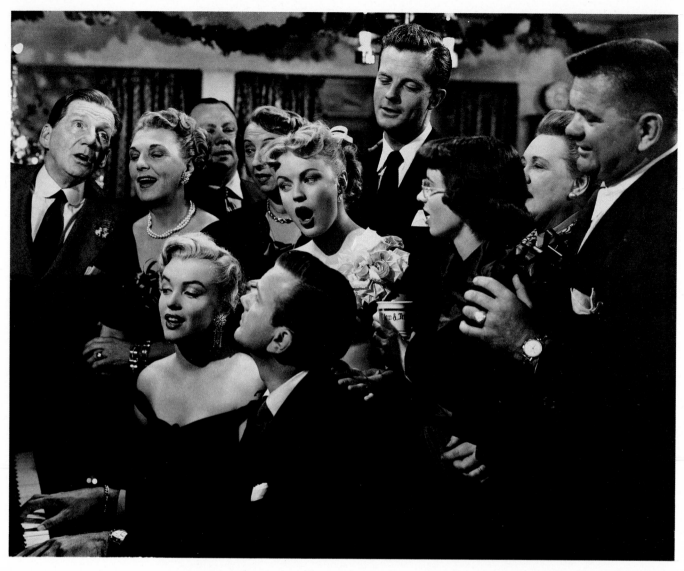

A June Haver film, *Love Nest*
(Twentieth Century-Fox),
provided a showcase for
Marilyn Monroe, seen at the
piano with William Lundigan,
with whom she resumed a
friendship, and his new wife,
June Haver, behind.

a tree. You know – like a cool drink when
you've got a fever.'

Miller, it seems, was similarly impressed.
He wrote to her about her relationship with
her public: 'Bewitch them with this image
they ask for, but I hope and almost pray you
won't be hurt in this game, nor ever change
... If you want someone to admire, why
not Abraham Lincoln? Carl Sandburg has
written a magnificent biography of him.'

Marilyn's next movie was *Love Nest*,
which was written by I. A. L. Diamond,
who was later, with Billy Wilder, to write
one of her greatest films, *Some Like It Hot*.
Love Nest, though, was a pretty tepid affair,
concerned as it was with the zany goings-on
in an apartment building arising from the
arrival of 'Bobby' (Monroe) to take up her
friendship again with hero William Lundigan
who is now happily married to June Haver.
After that, in 1951, there was *Let's Make It
Legal*, with Claudette Colbert and Macdonald Carey, about a couple seeking divorce.
It was about this time, as though taking the

title of that movie to heart, that Marilyn
decided to contact the man whom she believed was her real father. This man, whom
she thought from her mother's account to
have sired her, now owned a dairy farm, and
the film *Marilyn, The Untold Story* reveals
– how truthfully we do not know – that she
and Natasha Lytess drove out into the country to see him. On the way there, Marilyn
decided to phone him. She was told by a
secretary that he did not wish to speak to
her; any 'complaint' should be put in
writing.

That the incident occurred there can be
little doubt. But what was said is disputable.
Certainly, though, the fact that it happened
at all is indicative of the fact that at this stage
of her career – with all lines seemingly open
to her ambition – she desperately needed to
feel that she was rooted to something, even
if it were as illusory as an imagined father.
This feeling she was never to lose. At that
time, after a series of not very good movies
for Twentieth Century-Fox, she transmuted

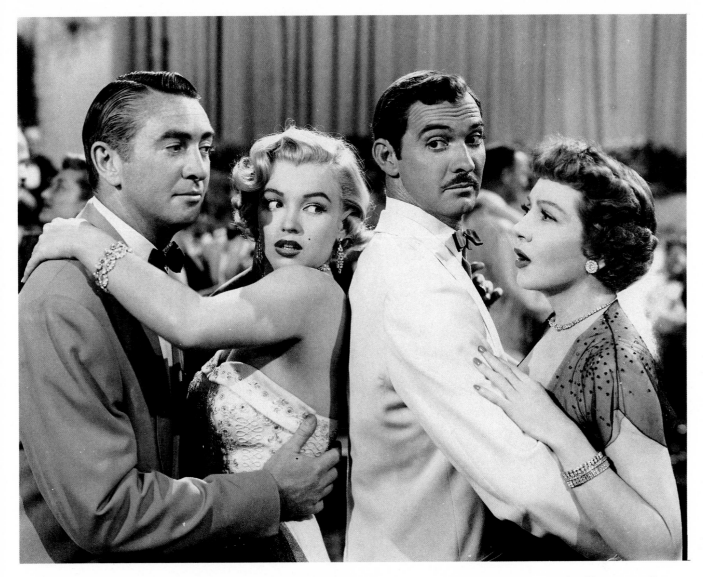

it into a realization that she needed more acting expertise. She was already working with Natasha Lytess ('I taught her how to walk, how to breathe') but she now consulted another acting coach, Michael Chekhov, who tested her out in 'King Lear' as Cordelia, and was impressed by the sensitivity and range which seemed to be at her command: 'She has an instinct which is quite astonishing; all she needs is the technique to bring that instinct out into the open.'

What came out into the open around this time were stills from the nude calendar that Marilyn posed for while still Norma Jean, pictures from a different life, a different time. The moralists made much of them – there were even leaders written in some of the mid-West papers wondering if this were the way somebody in the public eye should have behaved. To some extent such adverse publicity was defused by her role in *Clash by Night*, from a play by Clifford Odets. This, an everyday story of fishing folk, was about an explosive, adulterous relationship in a

small fish-canning town, with Marilyn as an innocently bewildered girl. Her performance in this excited the critics, although her co-stars – Paul Douglas, Barbara Stanwyck and Robert Ryan – were not themselves very happy with Marilyn's on-set behaviour while making the movie. Marilyn had now got into the habit, almost a ritual, of having Natasha Lytess accompany her on her forays into acting. During breaks they would hold whispered conferences on how best to approach the coming scene; it was not an approach that was always best appreciated by directors, who wanted to put their own style and stamp upon what was being filmed.

Marilyn was also becoming unpopular with her colleagues because of her unpunctuality. Although she would arrive in good time for the start of shooting, she would then spend an inordinately long time making up and preparing herself for the day's work. In its way it may have been a subconscious rebellion against her earlier years, especially at the orphanage, when she had been made to

Macdonald Carey, Marilyn, Zachary Scott and Claudette Colbert in *Let's Make It Legal* (Twentieth Century-Fox), a domestic brouhaha about a couple who want a divorce.

Keith Andes and Marilyn in *Clash by Night* (RKO Radio), during the making of which Marilyn's later much-publicized lateness and unpredictability on set caused problems, especially with stars Robert Ryan and Barbara Stanwyck.

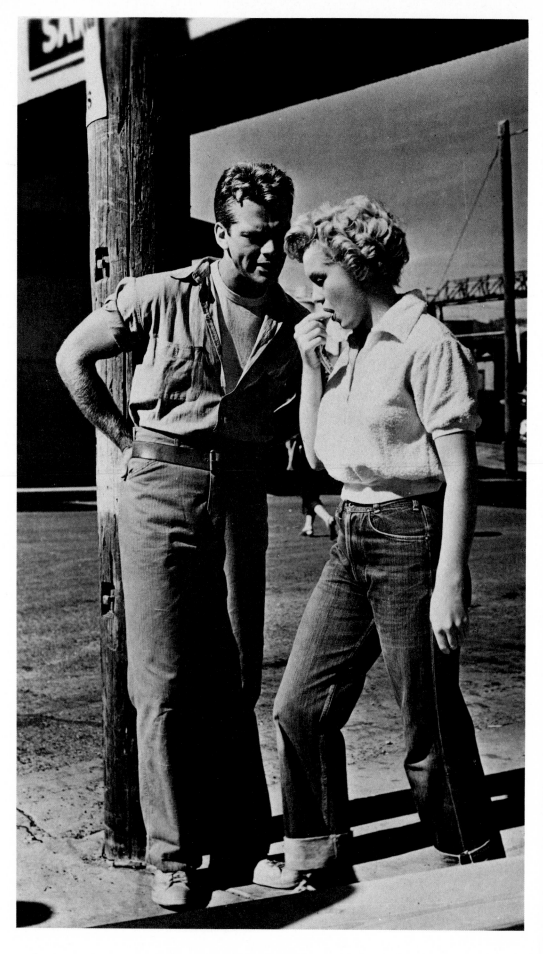

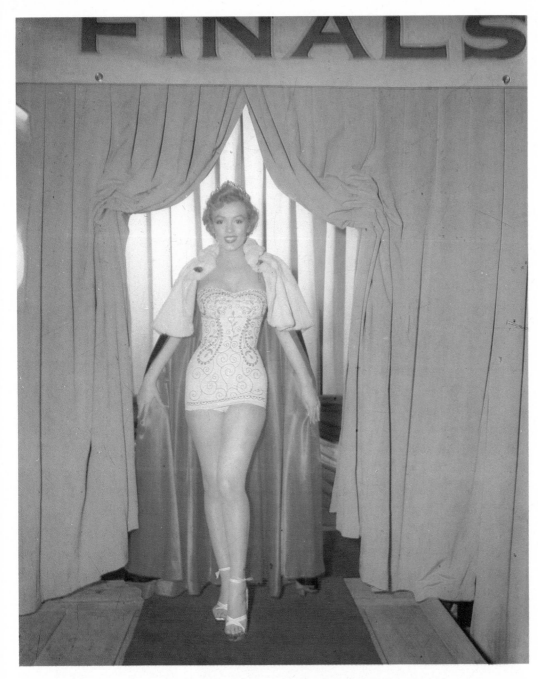

Marilyn in a 'Miss America' contest in *We're Not Married* (Twentieth Century-Fox), a comedy in which five married couples find that they aren't legally married at all, thus enabling Marilyn to switch from the 'Mrs America' contest.

live her life by other people's clocks. 'It was always up at a certain time,' she later recalled, 'go to bed at a certain time. Meals were set at a particular moment and if you were a minute late then you didn't get anything to eat. I hated all that.' That assertion of independence, though, at the studios, did not endear her to other professionals such as her actor-colleagues, who themselves realized that they had to work to other people's clocks – if only to ensure that the product came in on time. Robert Ryan was reported to have been particularly incensed: 'She just didn't seem to understand that we all relied upon each other.'

Despite these strictures, Marilyn was more than tolerated by the studio bosses, who were aware that they had a girl who was fast approaching the status of a star, a girl whom the public appreciated had that unique charisma which made her special. Not all her movies were accepted, though. *Don't Bother to Knock*, in 1952, was pretty much of a disaster in that it portrayed her as a neurotically disturbed baby-sitter in a large hotel, who is persuaded not to kill herself and her charge by Richard Widmark. It was not so much that she seemed very much out of character in the story, but that the whole was ill-conceived and badly managed in the way the narrative was eventually executed. More to everyone's taste around this time was *O. Henry's Full House*, an omnibus collection of short stories, in which she, as a vul-

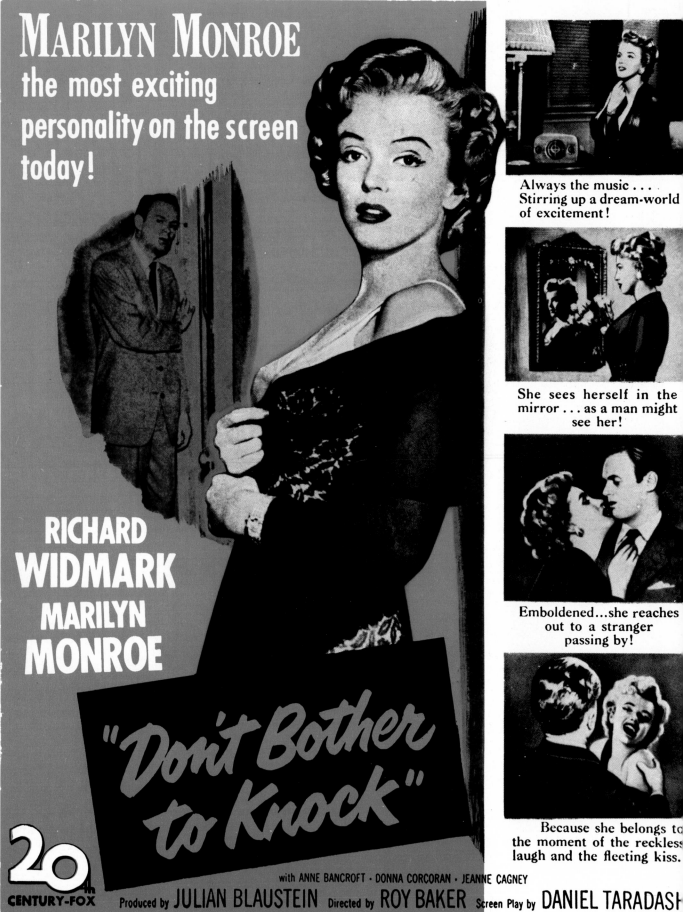

MARILYN MONROE
the most exciting personality on the screen today!

RICHARD WIDMARK
MARILYN MONROE

"*Don't Bother to Knock*"

20th CENTURY-FOX

with ANNE BANCROFT · DONNA CORCORAN · JEANNE CAGNEY

Produced by JULIAN BLAUSTEIN Directed by ROY BAKER Screen Play by DANIEL TARADASH

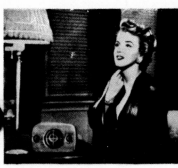

Always the music . . . Stirring up a dream-world of excitement!

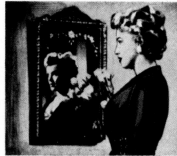

She sees herself in the mirror . . . as a man might see her!

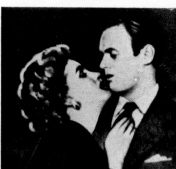

Emboldened...she reaches out to a stranger passing by!

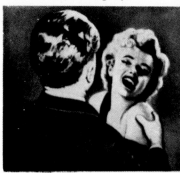

Because she belongs to the moment of the reckless laugh and the fleeting kiss.

32

nerable young prostitute, was teamed with Charles Laughton. Laughton was considered a dramatic wonder-worker, and Marilyn later said: 'It was like being in the presence of God.' Laughton, however, was charm itself and he, too, was later to talk about Marilyn's 'marvellous instinct and ability to project herself in front of the camera'.

More comically she was, too, to make *Monkey Business* with Cary Grant, Irene Dunne and Charles Coburn, a whimsy which recounts the shenanigans which occur when an elixir of youth gets mixed in with the water cooler – and everyone reverts to juvenilia. This was followed, at about the beginning of 1953, by *Niagara,* directed by Henry Hathaway, with Marilyn as the

would-be erring wife married to a sombre older man, Joseph Cotten. It was not, as a movie, very successful in what it set out to do, but the box-office receipts were good and the studio bosses were delighted that the contract with Marilyn was working well.

Fox was now teaming Marilyn with other beautiful stars. She played alongside Jane Russell in *Gentlemen Prefer Blondes,* which was an overblown musical based on the witty book by Anita Loos, with Marilyn as an eye-catching, mindboggling gold-digger, Lorelei. Archer Winsten in the *New York Post* said: 'The picture, not content with good-enough, broadens an already broad theme, thereby coming too close to burlesque for constant satisfaction.'

Left: Marilyn received scathing notices for *Don't Bother to Knock* (Twentieth Century-Fox), in which, despite the showcard, the glamour-girl role was replaced by a difficult acting one – Marilyn was a psychopathic baby-sitter planning to murder her charge.

Below: *O. Henry's Full House* (Twentieth Century-Fox) was a collection of five stories, in one of which, 'The Cop and the Anthem', Marilyn played a streetwalker opposite Charles Laughton.

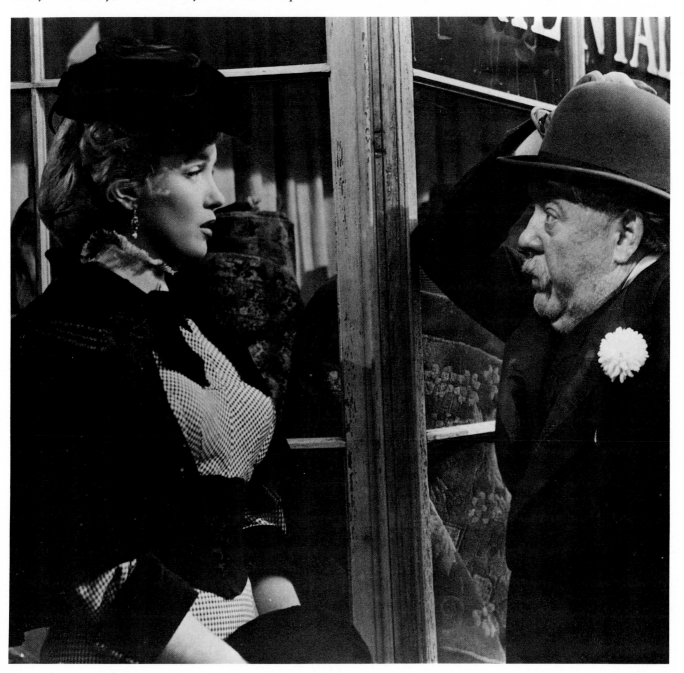

Marilyn had a starring role in *Niagara* (Twentieth Century-Fox) and became ever more famous as a sex queen as she wore tight outfits which made every walk away from the camera into an exciting spectacle.

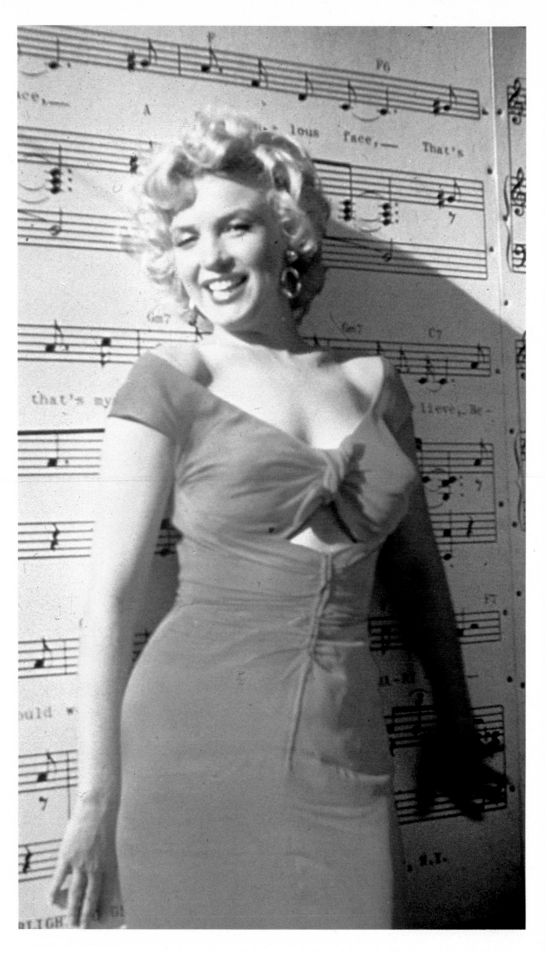

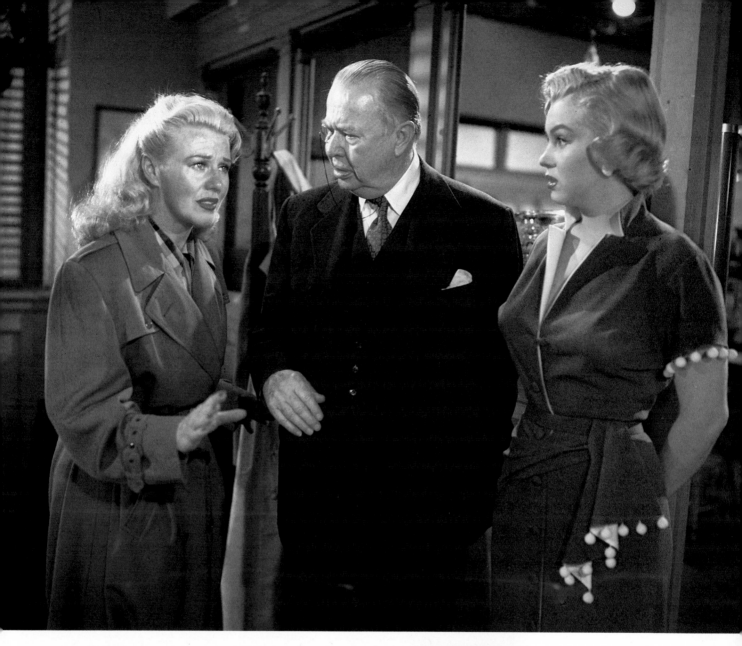

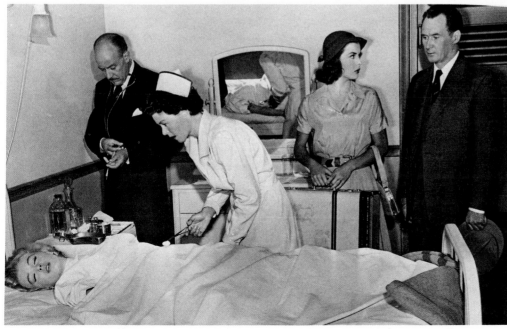

Above: *Monkey Business* (Twentieth Century-Fox) was a comedy in which Cary Grant took a youth elixir and turned into a baby. Charles Coburn and his secretary Marilyn listen as a distraught Ginger Rogers, as Grant's wife, relates the story.

Left: Marilyn tries to have her husband, Joseph Cotton, killed in *Niagara* (Twentieth Century-Fox) and at one point almost achieves her own screen demise.

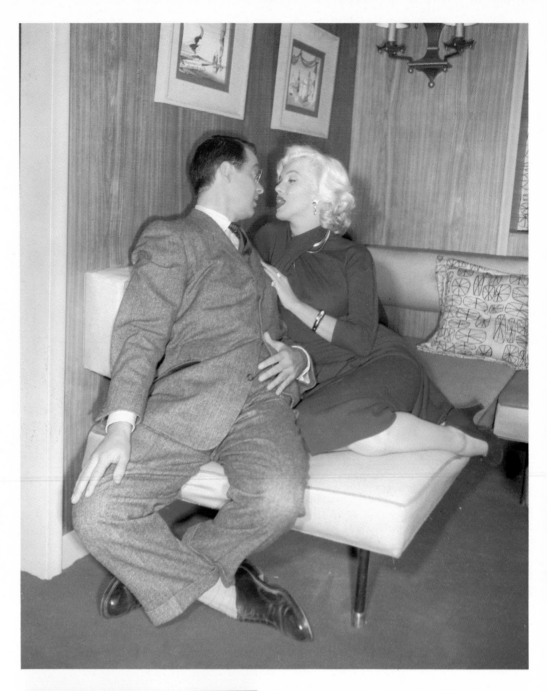

Far right: All big girls together. Marilyn and Jane Russell in *Gentlemen Prefer Blondes* (Twentieth Century-Fox). Marilyn was Lorelei, the silly and seductive blonde from Anita Loos' best-selling book.

Right: Blondes also seem to prefer gentlemen. Marilyn making up to Elliott Reid in *Gentlemen Prefer Blondes* (Twentieth Century-Fox).

Right: Marilyn off the set of *Gentlemen Prefer Blondes*, with her famous director Howard Hawks.

Overleaf: The second 1953 film in which Marilyn played a gold-digger, *How to Marry a Millionaire* (Twentieth Century-Fox). She is dreaming of receiving all the crown jewels from her millionaire boyfriend Alex D'Arcy.

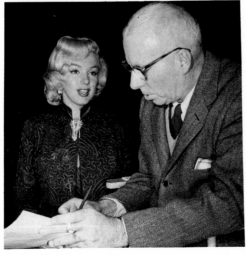

After that there was *How to Marry a Millionaire* with Betty Grable and Lauren Bacall, again about gold-diggers looking for rich husbands. This was more stylish, and Archer Winsten redeemed himself in Marilyn's eyes by writing that it was 'an extremely entertaining film'. Its box-office success helped massage her ego, too.

Personally, Marilyn was now considered something of a hermit; she had partially broken off her friendship with Natasha Lytess for some reason which is still obscure, and occupied herself with other close, personal friends. She was brought out of that darkness, though, by the man she was to marry and whom in a way she was to love for the rest of her life: Joe DiMaggio.

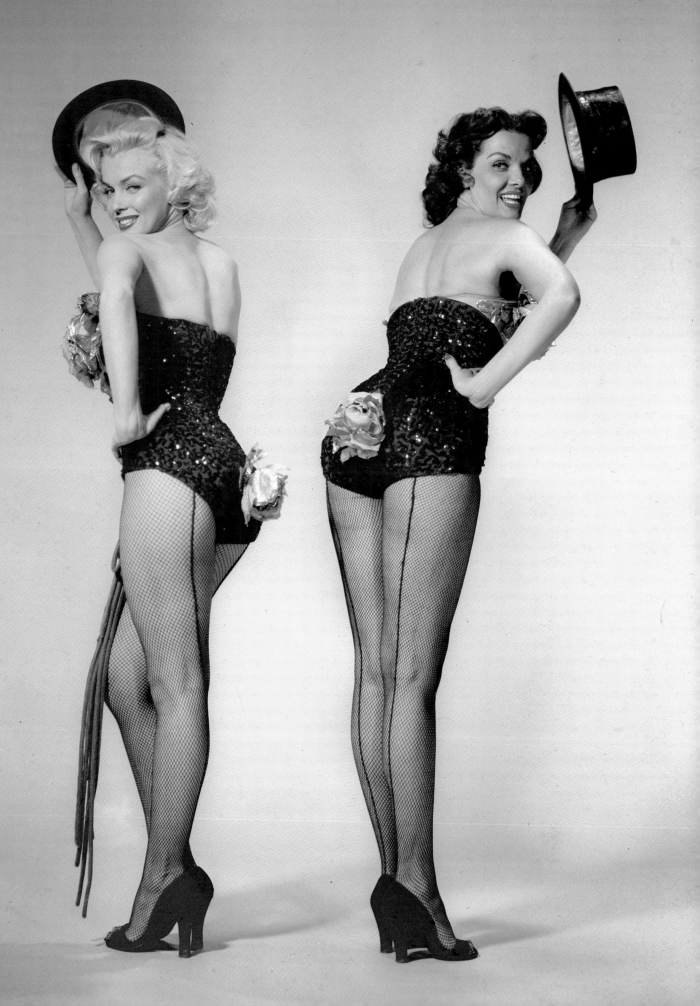

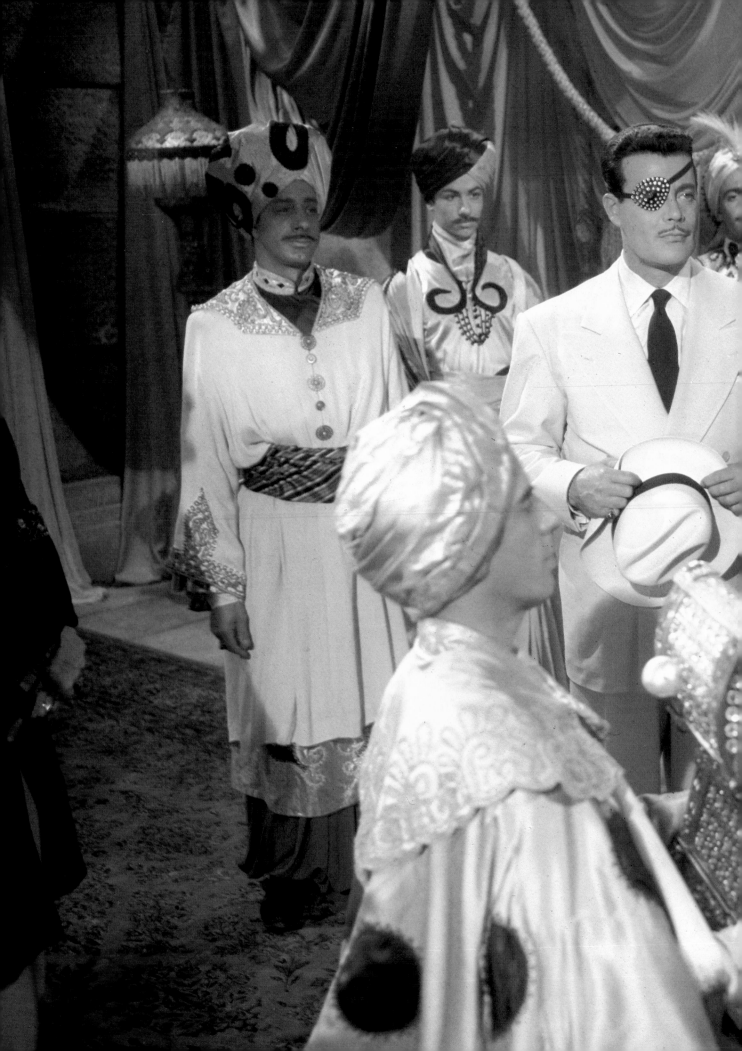

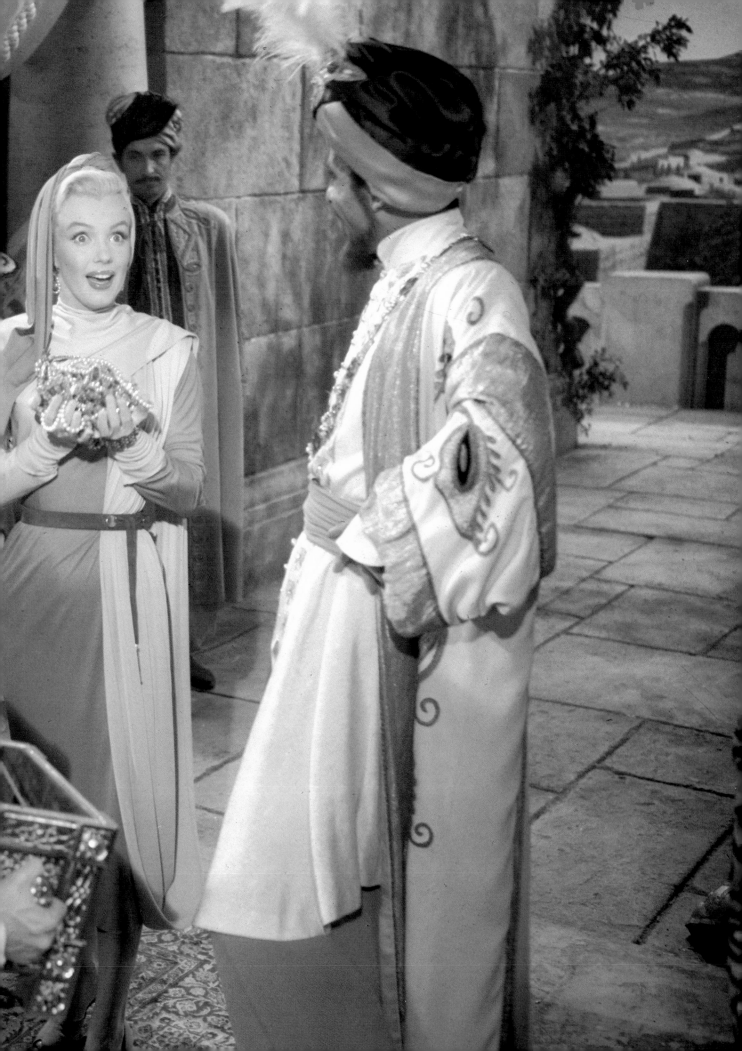

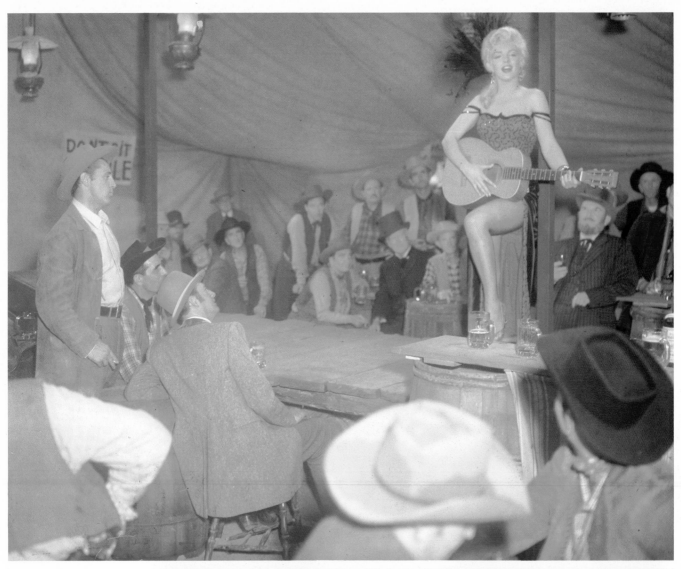

Above: Robert Mitchum, on the left, sizes up the dance-hall entertainer, played by Marilyn, in *River of No Return* (Twentieth Century-Fox), a rugged outdoor film shot on location in Canada.

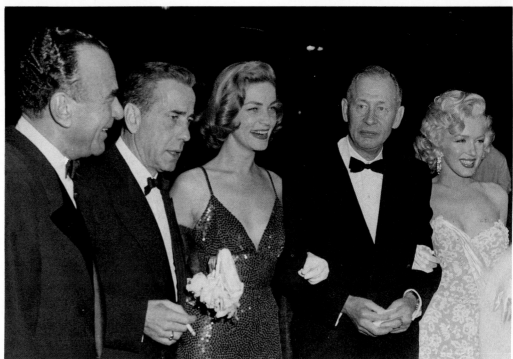

Right: Marilyn at the premiere in 1953 of *How to Marry a Millionaire*. With her, from the left, are George Bowser, Humphrey Bogart, Lauren Bacall and Nunnally Johnson.

40

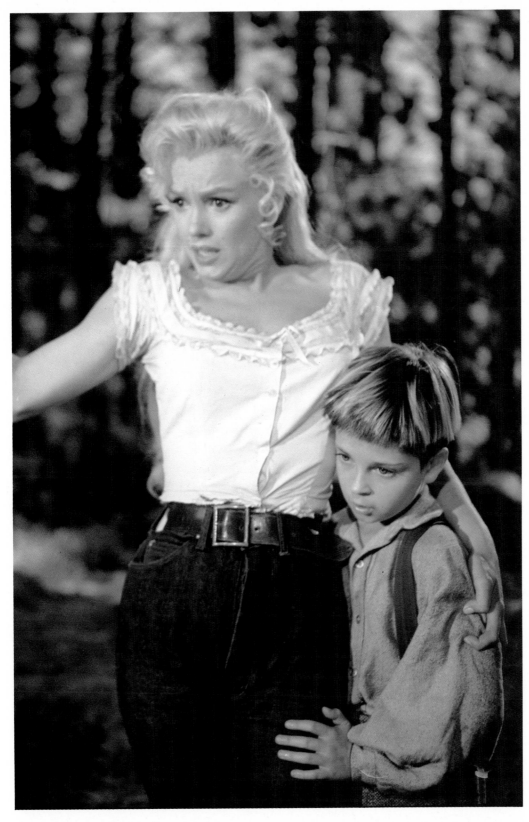

The reason for the horror shown by Marilyn and little Tommy Rettig in *River of No Return* (Twentieth Century-Fox) is a battle between Robert Mitchum, without his gun, and a mountain lion, on their flight through the northwest frontier wilderness.

She met him before she went on to make *River of No Return* for Otto Preminger. A double dating had been arranged, but she had forgotten all about it, arriving more than an hour later when reminded of its existence. At that time DiMaggio was the most famous baseball player in America, but Marilyn was not particularly interested in that, so conceivably she took him on first sight and as he was 'like a businessman, he looked so conservative; I expected sportsmen to be much flashier than he turned out to be.' It was a friendship that lasted some months, before it became marriage, but it brought

Marilyn out into the world again.

So much so that she was able to fight back when the irascible Otto Preminger ordered Natasha Lytess off the set of *River of No Return:* Marilyn went immediately to Darryl F. Zanuck and Natasha was partially reinstated. It shows something of the power that Marilyn realized she could wield, that she went straight to the studio boss – and that he agreed with her rather than the more senior Preminger. The film itself is no great shakes, with Marilyn as a deserted wife (!) hiring Robert Mitchum to bring back her husband. But it works well in terms of its own simple narrative. Nevertheless, Marilyn was not happy with the kind of movies she was making at Twentieth Century-Fox and, with photographer Milton Greene and his wife, Amy, set up herself as her own company. That was on the professional side of her life; on the private side was her marriage to Joe DiMaggio, on 14 January 1954.

The wedding took place in San Francisco's City Hall with Marilyn wearing a fashionable, but conservative, brown suit at DiMaggio's request. The spectators were many and inquisitive. Everyone had eyes for Marilyn, but she only had eyes for DiMaggio. 'I may even retire,' she told the Pressmen. 'I may just do that.'

Marilyn kissing the man she probably loved most in her life, Joe DiMaggio, after their wedding in 1954.

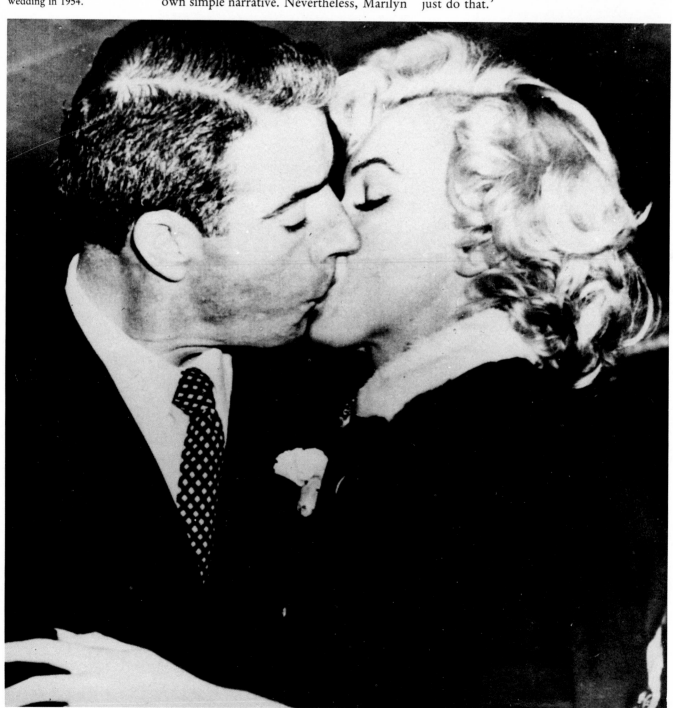

A SUPERSTAR IS BORN

The first stop of Marilyn's and DiMaggio's honeymoon was Honolulu, the second was Tokyo. In both places DiMaggio became aware of just what kind of legend he had married. Mobs of fans ran screaming at the two of them – security had not been alerted – and the DiMaggios had literally to run for cover. DiMaggio was later to say it was the most frightening experience of his life. Marilyn, too, was reported as saying that she was terrified, but in a way it was an experience that was to help her in her by now antagonistic dealings with Twentieth Century-Fox. They had sent her a script of *The Girl in Pink Tights,* the script which she regarded as 'lousy', and rejected. The studio thought this was just a tactic to upgrade her contract and threatened action. The reports coming in from afar now made them realize that Marilyn was not just any actress to be kicked around at their discretion; she was, in every sense, a superstar, whose charisma crossed all frontiers, barriers and languages.

This realization was made even more evident when she decided she wanted to entertain the American troops fighting in North Korea. DiMaggio at first argued against it, but she won him over to her point of view and Marilyn made what can only be described as a conquest. Occasionally, there were what were reported to be 'small riots' among the soldiers anticipating her arrival. She sang, she danced, she generally cavorted for them, in all ways living up to the sexy Barbie Doll image that the studios, and to some extent she herself, had created. A writer in the *New York Times* complained that the troops had rioted wildly 'and behaved like bobby-soxers in Times Square, not like soldiers proud of their uniform'. But if Marilyn's appearances had raised temperatures, either with indignation or sensuality, she herself succumbed more physically on her way back to Tokyo and contracted a kind of mild pneumonia. It took her some days to recover, and then she and DiMaggio toured the rest of Japan. After all, they were still on honeymoon.

Then it was back to Twentieth Century-Fox and into her next movie – not *Pink*

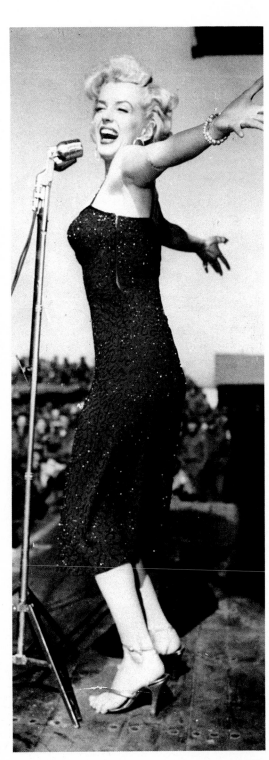

On her honeymoon with DiMaggio, Marilyn stopped off to entertain troops fighting in Korea. It was against DiMaggio's wishes and he was taken aback by the adulation and applause she received.

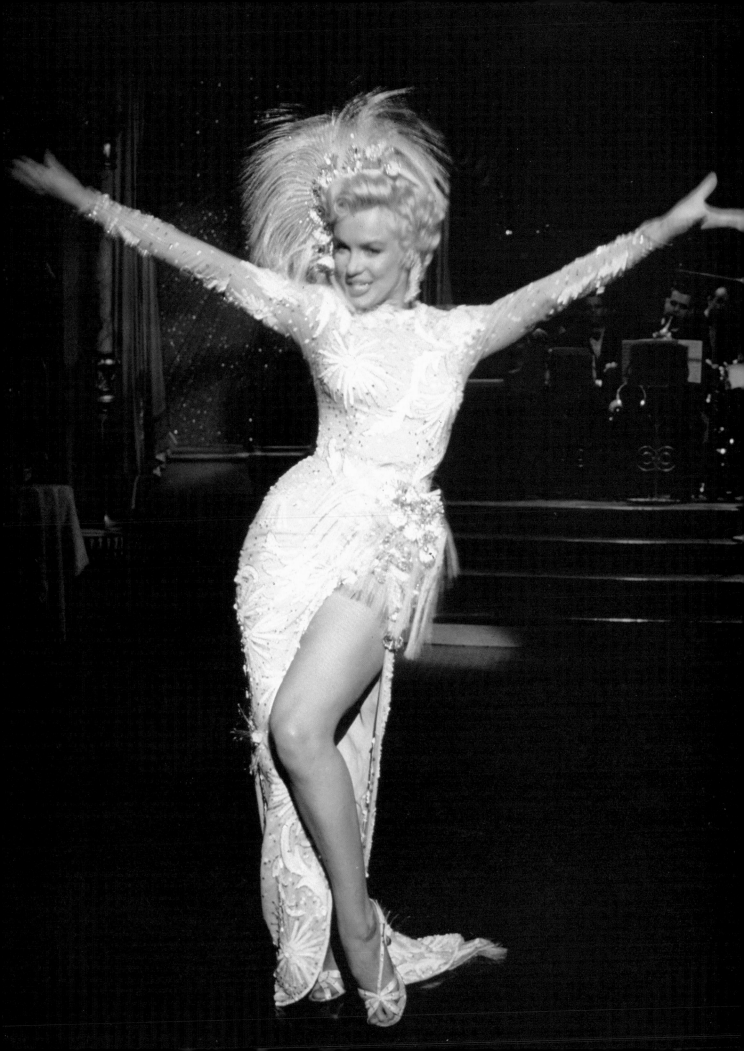

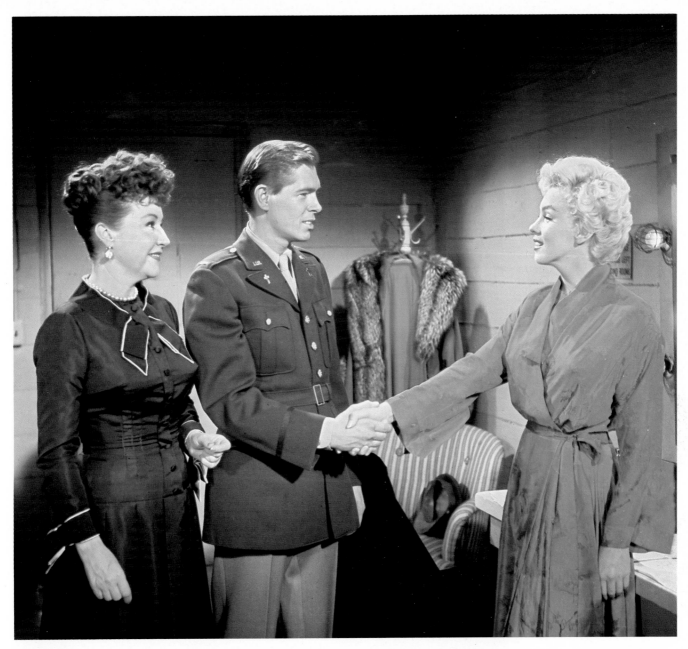

Tights, but *There's No Business like Show Business*, a curious amalgam of schmaltz and absurdity with Marilyn as a sexy singer of saucy songs. She sang three numbers, 'After You Get What You Want You Don't Want It', 'Heat Wave', and 'Lazy'. It had a mixed reception from the critics. Bosley Crowther, of the *New York Times*, who had previously been an admirer of Marilyn's work, lamented her 'wriggling and squirming . . . which are embarrassing to behold'. But Frank Quinn of the *New York Daily Mirror* described her performance as 'sizzling'. You paid your money and you took your choice.

Marilyn's next film-choice was to be, in 1955, *The Seven Year Itch*, co-written by Billy Wilder, who also directed. It was a day-dream fantasy with Tom Ewell, without his wife for the summer, as the middle-aged

husband fantasizing about The Girl (Marilyn) who has moved into an adjoining compartment. It became famous, not to say notorious, for one scene in which Marilyn, standing above an air-vent in the road, has her flounced skirt blown high.

The occasion was filmed on location in New York and Joe DiMaggio came along, too. That he was dismayed by the sexy way his wife seemed to be displaying herself has been well noted. During the scene with the skirt flying upwards, watched by a crowd of people who had heard that the film was in production, he stood and watched with distaste. One newspaper reporter asked him: 'What do you think of Marilyn having to show more of herself than she's shown before, Joe?' DiMaggio did not answer directly, but walked away, his views evident

Above: *There's No Business like Show Business* (Twentieth Century-Fox), and Ethel Merman introduces her priest son, Johnnie Ray, to Marilyn.

Left: Marilyn oomphing it up in another scene from *There's No Business like Show Business* (Twentieth Century-Fox) as she does justice to her torrid dress and Irving Berlin's songs.

in every taut line of his body. This incident plus what had happened in North Korea, Japan and Honolulu led DiMaggio to feel that he had had enough of being married to an institution that was as much part of the national consciousness as the Statue of Liberty. Returning to Hollywood, he and Marilyn announced that they were separating, to divorce. Later, in 1961, it was reported that they were dating again. But then and there in 1955 it was very definitely over, and Marilyn returned to shooting on *The Seven Year Itch*.

The premiere and the resulting box-office returns of the movie proved that it was a smash-hit, and on the strength of it she was able to negotiate a contract giving her script and director approval for the future. Her private life may have been a mess – she was now going to a psychoanalyst five times a week besides taking acting lessons at Lee and Paula Strasberg's famous Actors' Studio – but her public life was being structured with some success. Bosley Crowther returned to the fold of her fan club and wrote of *The Seven Year Itch:* 'Miss Monroe brings a special personality and certain physical something or other to the film that may not be exactly what the playwright ordered, but which definitely conveys an idea.

Right: The famous scene from *The Seven Year Itch* (Twentieth Century-Fox) in which Marilyn's dress is blown up by the air from a subway grating. Many watched the shooting with enjoyment, but husband Joe DiMaggio was disturbed at the way his wife was being displayed.

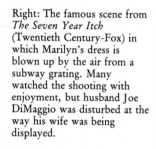

Far right: Tom Ewell as a husband alone and Marilyn Monroe as the kinky girl upstairs trying to cool off on a sweltering day but raising Ewell's temperature instead in the hilarious smash *The Seven Year Itch* (Twentieth Century-Fox).

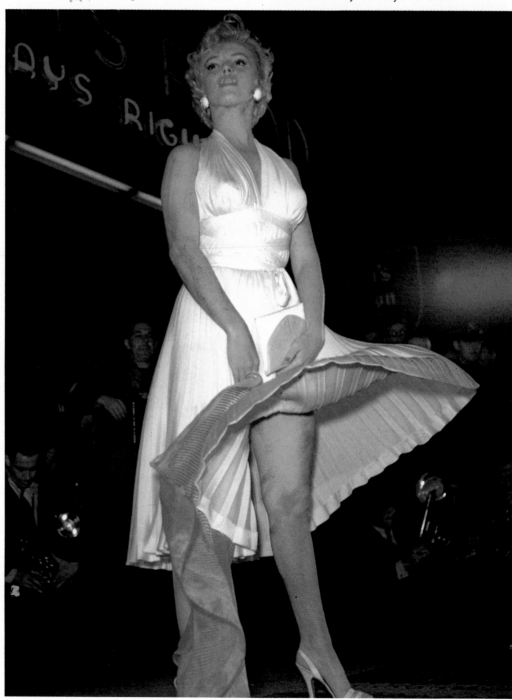

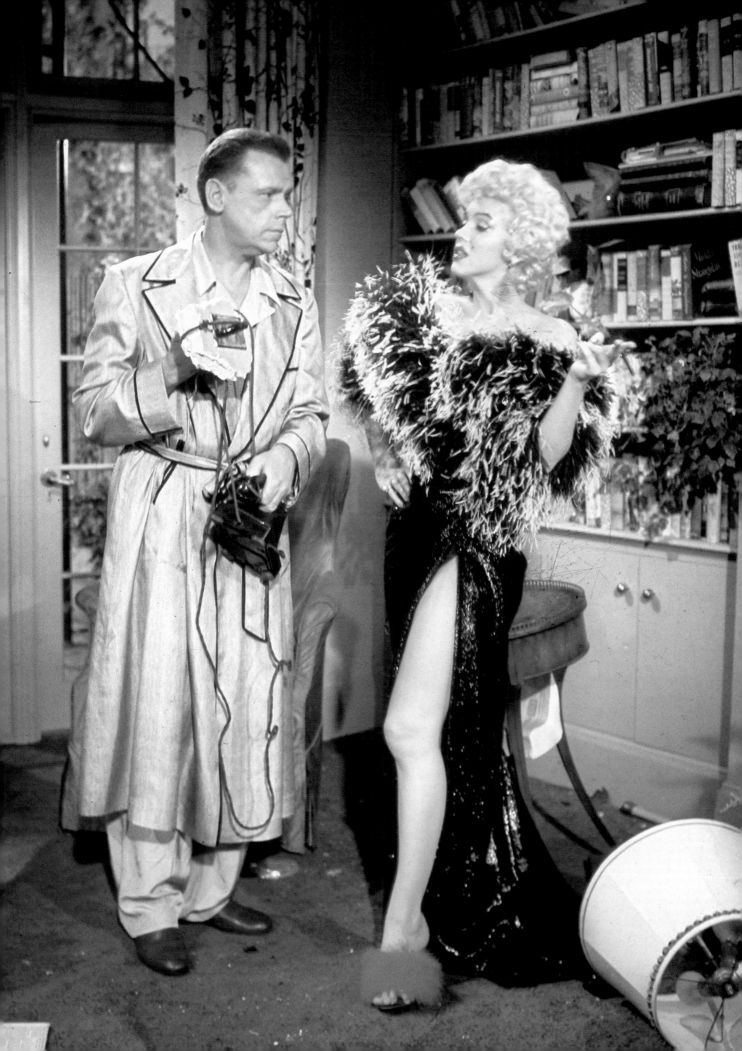

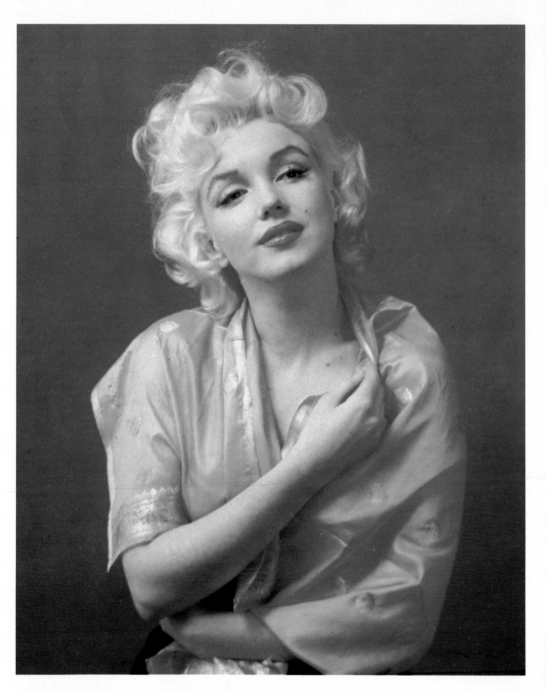

The mature Marilyn, without the slinky dresses and the over-coiffured hair, sometimes conveyed a winsome quality more attractive than her ultra-glamorous image.

'From the moment she steps into the picture, in a garment that drapes her shapely form as though she had been skilfully poured into it, the famous screen star with the silver-blonde tresses and ingenuously wide-eyed stare emanates one suggestion. And that suggestion rather dominates the film. It is – well, why define it? Miss Monroe clearly plays the title role.'

It was about this time, late in 1955, that Marilyn met again the playwright Arthur Miller, with whom she had become friendly before her marriage to Joe DiMaggio. It seemed to her to be an inevitable furtherance of her 'intellectualization' process, which had attracted her to the Strasberg studio and which constantly made her try to define why

she acted in the way that she did, constantly looking for a purpose and meaning in a life which – despite her success – sometimes seemed meaningless to her. Part of this process was to be her next film, *Bus Stop*, which some critics consider her finest; certainly it was one of the most careful and reasoned of her roles so far. If she was once again playing a bit of a slut, at least it was a slut who had rhymes and reasons for being the way she was and whose hard glamour concealed an innocent heart.

William Inge's play, transmuted to film, is about a naive cowboy (Don Murray) who sees an 'angel' (Marilyn) singing in a night-club and thinks of her tawdriness as beatific. He virtually kidnaps her to take her back

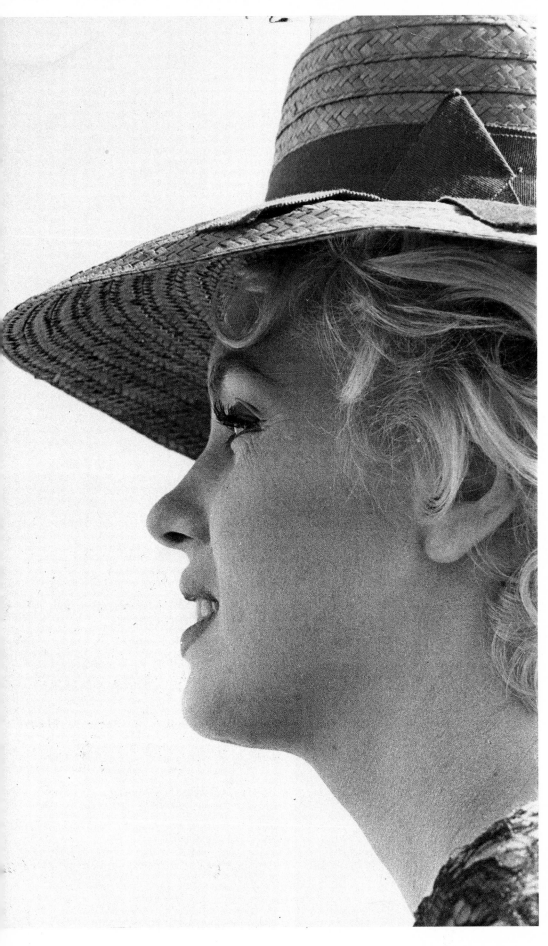

The sort of face one wouldn't mind standing next to at a bus stop. Marilyn in *Bus Stop* (Twentieth Century-Fox) was approaching 30, and there were small lines round her eyes, but she was no less beautiful.

Below: Marilyn looking as appealing as ever in *Bus Stop* (Twentieth Century-Fox) despite her cheap, tinselly dress.

home with him, and it is their coming together as personalities that forms the substance of the film. Josh Logan, who had a considerable reputation for coping with difficult stars, was the director, and all seemed set for what would be a rewarding experience. But Marilyn herself, as though realizing that her dramatic experience was at stake, was more nervous than she could ever remember being. Josh Logan had sent word that he did not want her dramatic coach, Paula Strasberg, on set, and she felt deprived and bereft of sympathetic companionship. She all but alienated her co-star, Don Murray, when she hit him harder than need be, during a scene when she is supposed to flick him with part of her dress. He walked off, but later relented because of Marilyn's abject apologies and came back. The film-making was a chapter of minor incidents, including a bout of bronchitis for Marilyn, which meant that Logan had to 'shoot around' her. Later she was to berate him for cutting out what she thought were her most exciting moments, but at the time she basked in the glow of critical approval. Bosley Crowther, of the *New York Times,* was typical of the

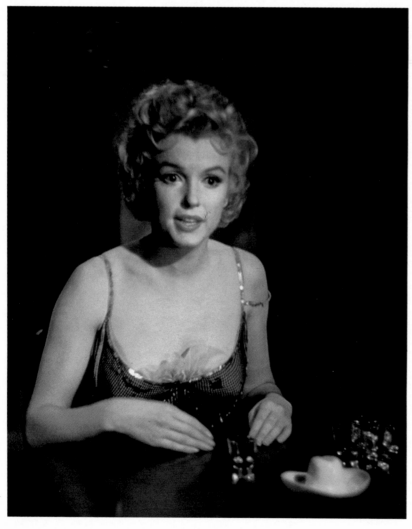

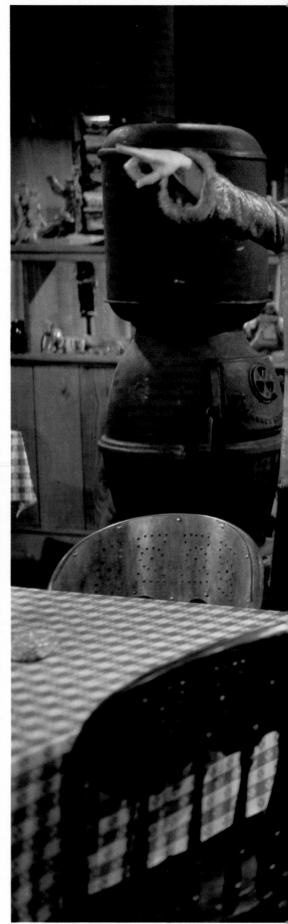

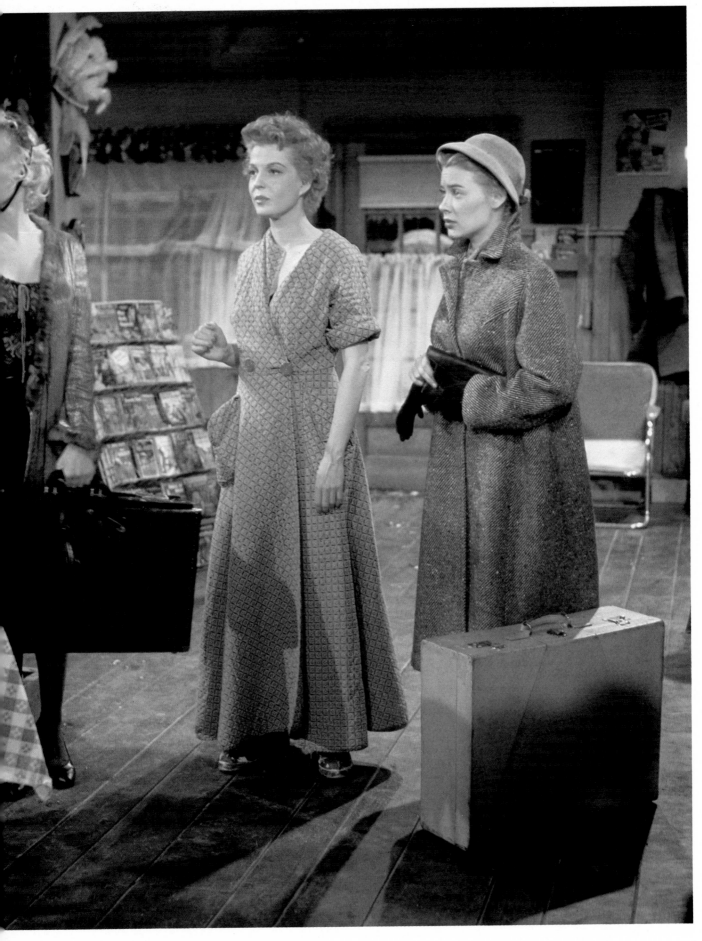

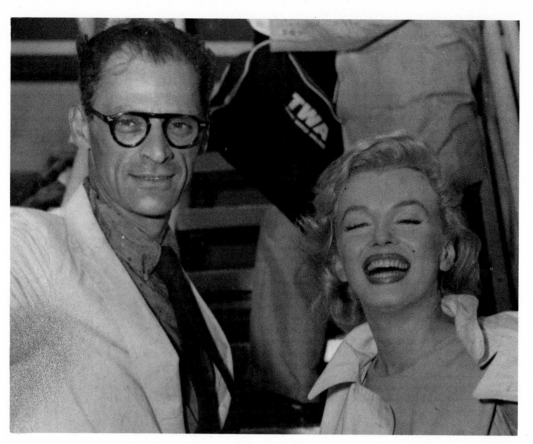

Marilyn and new husband Arthur Miller leave Idlewild Airport in New York for a honeymoon in England. Miller had passport difficulties, and they were summoned to appear as witnesses to a fatal road accident on their wedding day, but eventually left on time.

many: 'Hold on to your chairs, everybody, and get set for a rattling surprise. Marilyn Monroe has finally proved herself an actress in *Bus Stop*. She and the picture are swell!' And William K. Zinsser, of the *New York Herald Tribune*, wrote: 'In *Bus Stop* she has a wonderful role and she plays it with a mixture of humour and pain that is very touching. This is also the special genius of the movie. One minute it is uproariously funny, the next minute tender and fragile, and somehow Josh Logan preserves the delicate balance.'

All of which must have been pleasing for the girl who had been trying to learn to act, to rationalize the instinct she had for projection. Even more to delight in was the fact that she and Arthur Miller had finally decided to get married after his divorce. He was having some trouble with his passport, because the current climate of political harassment in America implied that he had Communist leanings, but when that was sorted out all would be well.

Certainly all became well in that direction, but another dilemma now faced the couple. Miller was Jewish: should Marilyn become Jewish? It took time but eventually that was accomplished. Nothing seemed to stand in their way, nor did it. In June 1956 Marilyn Monroe and Arthur Miller were married in a Jewish double-ring ceremony after an earlier civil wedding. In its way it was a

symbolic occasion. Miller stood for the intellectual side of the American dream, Marilyn for the physical. By coming together as man and wife two halves became a whole, a sphere of unity which Marilyn's American public recognized as entirely appropriate for their idol. It was an indication of the status that she had attained, of the fact that she was taken seriously as an actress.

Her next venture, though, was to cast her down from those heights of elation. It was to be a film that would be of her own choosing and it was to be with Britain's finest actor: Laurence Olivier. Its title was *The Prince and the Showgirl*.

Marilyn Monroe Productions had been set up with the help of Milton Greene, but Marilyn herself was doubly dubious about what the company's first movie should be. Then she read the script of the play written by the British playwright, Terence Rattigan, and decided that this was for her: the role of Elsie, the chorus girl in the London of 1911 who becomes involved with the Prince Regent (Olivier) of Carpathia and his son who is about to become the king (Jeremy Spenser). She and Miller decided to travel to England for the production and their first public meeting with Olivier was cordial in the extreme.

Neither Marilyn nor Miller knew that Olivier had been making enquiries of his friend Josh Logan about what Marilyn was like to work with. Olivier liked the reported witticisms of which Marilyn was capable – 'What did you have on?' 'The radio' – and thought that that humour would come through in *The Prince and the Showgirl*, which he would produce as well as direct. Logan assured him that if coaxed she could be a real trouper and was rarely late on set. Both Marilyn and Olivier having been assured of each other's credentials, the filming started. It was to be Marilyn's 25th film.

Whatever the reasons, on the set Marilyn began, observers noted, not so much acting as acting up. Some said that it was because of Olivier's strangely ham-fisted approach to her, antagonizing her especially when, during one difficult take, he commanded her to 'Look sexy, Marilyn!' This threw Marilyn back once more to the inmost realization that she was nothing more to some people, of whom Olivier appeared to be one, than a cinematic sex object. So she started being late on set. She was taken curiously ill. Arthur Miller bore the brunt of the unsaid accusa-

tions that Marilyn was really throwing a tantrum. It was Sybil Thorndike, *grande dame* of the British theatre, who really knew how to handle Marilyn. During one of her absences word reached Marilyn via Miller from her: 'Please ask her when she can come to the set. We all need her so desperately. She's the only one of us who can really act for the camera.' Marilyn went; this was coaxing which she really understood.

Shooting struggled on and was eventually completed after many arguments and rows; it was during this period that Marilyn also had a difference of opinion with Milton Greene which seemed to suggest that Marilyn Monroe Productions might soon be on the way out. Certainly Marilyn's public parting from Olivier did not seem to be as cordial as their first meeting. Years afterwards she said about her experience in Britain: 'It seemed to be raining the whole time. Or maybe it was me.'

Whatever it was, there was a deal of mixed criticism of *The Prince and the Showgirl*.

In *The Prince and the Showgirl* (Warner Brothers), Marilyn played the showgirl opposite Laurence Olivier's prince. Here they leave for the Coronation, accompanied by Richard Wattis and Sybil Thorndike.

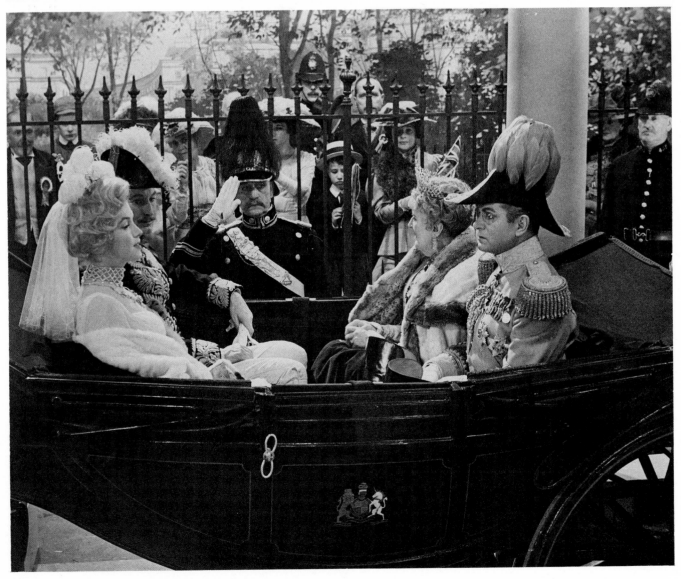

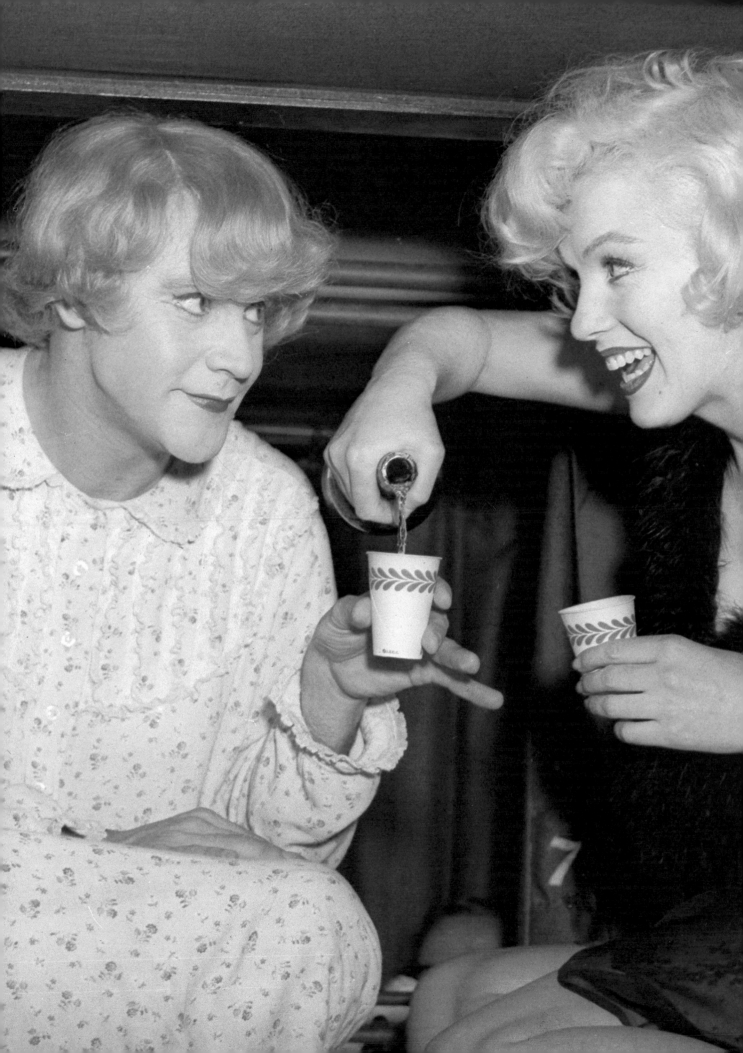

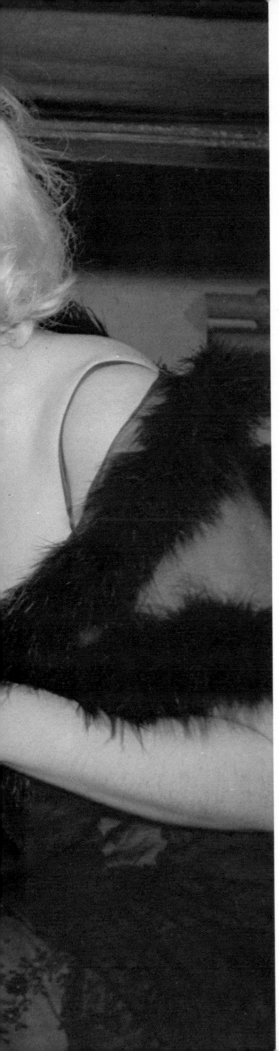

William K. Zinsser, of the *New York Herald Tribune*, while praising Olivier's performance, wrote: 'Marilyn's role had no such fine shadings. This is a dumb, affable showgirl and nothing more, and Miss Monroe goes through the motions with mirth, childish innocence, squeals of pleasure, pouts of annoyance, eyes big as golf balls and many a delighted toss of her rounded surfaces.' Which was as final a nail as any to knock into the coffin of what had not been a very happy experience at all. But that experience was only a prelude to the unhappiness she experienced in making a film which can nevertheless be ranked among her greatest, an all-time classic of comedy which can still be run and re-run and make audiences laugh all this time after its production in 1959: *Some Like It Hot.*

Director Billy Wilder's screenplay with I. A. L. Diamond was a spoof of the 1929 gangster era, with Jack Lemmon and Tony Curtis as two musicians who flee from hoodlums and end up with a girl band, which includes Marilyn as Sugar Kane, the ukelele player and singer with the orchestra. That Lemmon and Curtis are obliged to dress up as women and then find themselves constantly allured by the girls with whom they work is part of the joke, and Marilyn's performance as Sugar emerges as a delightful, self-mocking parody of sensuality. The whole works with the precision of Feydeau farce.

The production itself, though, did not work out like that. Wilder at one point blamed drama coach Paula Strasberg, whom Marilyn insisted on having on the set. Later he said about Marilyn: 'There has never been a woman with such voltage on the screen, with the exception of Garbo.' But that was with hindsight and with the affection of nostalgia.

At the time he said: 'The question is whether Marilyn is a person at all or one of the greatest DuPont products ever invented. She has breasts like granite; she defies gravity; and has a brain like Swiss cheese – full of holes. She hasn't the vaguest conception of the time of day. She arrives late and tells you she couldn't find the studio and she's been working there for years. There are certain wonderful rascals in this world, like Monroe, and one day they lie down on an analyst's couch and out comes a clenched dreary thing. It's better for Monroe not to be straightened out. The charm of her is her two left feet.'

Certainly her late arrivals on set, her constant consultations with Paula Strasberg and her fluffing of lines upset both Lemmon and Curtis. Lemmon was more discreet in his anger than Curtis, who was reported to have

An illicit drink on the train for Marilyn and Jack Lemmon in *Some Like It Hot* (United Artists). Lemmon and Tony Curtis are runaway musicians who to escape hoodlums dress as girls and join an all-female band.

55

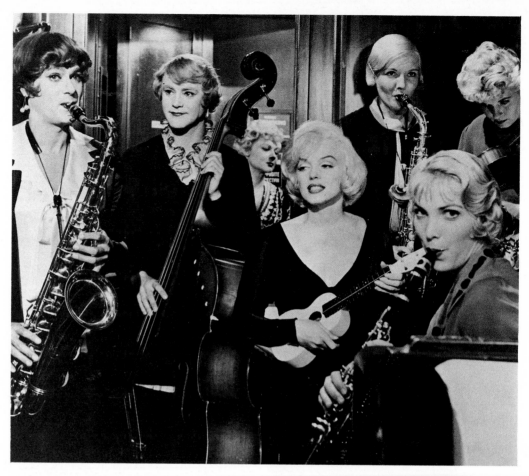

Right: All girls together in *Some Like It Hot* (United Artists). Tony Curtis and Jack Lemmon as pretty unlikely-looking girls and the undoubted genuine article, Marilyn, playing her more modest instrument.

Far right: Another picture of the 'girls' from *Some Like It Hot* (United Artists). Marilyn is the one with the ladder in her tights.

said later that kissing Marilyn was 'like kissing Hitler'. Whether or not Marilyn's contrariness in coping with her fellow-stars and Wilder himself may have had something to do with a recent miscarriage it's hard to say. She told her maid Lena Pepitone that just because she was in another comedy it wouldn't prevent her from becoming a serious dramatic actress someday . . . she wanted to have a real career. She wanted to act, to have friends, to be happy. She wanted some respect, not to be laughed at, and feared that others misunderstood her.

She was very aware that she was too fat in the movie and kept saying so all the way through the eventual premiere. She felt that the audience was laughing *at* and not with the film itself. It was a gruelling experience for her, and one that was only made more happy by the critical reviews. The American trade paper *Variety* called *Some Like It Hot* 'the funniest picture of recent memory . . . Marilyn has never looked better. Her performance as "Sugar", the fuzzy blonde who likes saxophone players and men with glasses has a deliciously naive quality. She's a comedienne with that combination of sex appeal and timing that just can't be beat.'

Billy Wilder was asked in an interview if he would go through the experience again and said: 'I have discussed this with my doc-

tor and my psychiatrist and they tell me I'm too old and too rich to go through this again.' Arthur Miller demanded an apology on Marilyn's behalf, but didn't get one. The atmosphere between Wilder and Miller was frigid until they met again around two years later. Then they made it up.

Marilyn's relationship with Arthur Miller, though, was deteriorating. It would survive some time longer, but she and he found that they were steadily drifting apart. Then, along came her next film, *Let's Make Love*, and a French leading man, Yves Montand, with whom she felt more at peace and at ease than she had with any man for a long time. Montand had brought his actress wife, Simone Signoret, with him, but that did not deter the sparks that flew between Marilyn and him. She told Lena Pepitone: 'You should see him, Lena. He's great. Imagine if Joe DiMaggio could sing. That's what he's like.' That Yves Montand was in the film at all was because American actors such as Gregory Peck had turned the script down. It wasn't, as she thought, that they didn't want to act with her, it was just that the script was adjudged awful.

Marilyn, however, had some faith in it – especially in Montand – and decided they would go ahead. It was a decision that did nobody any good at all.

56

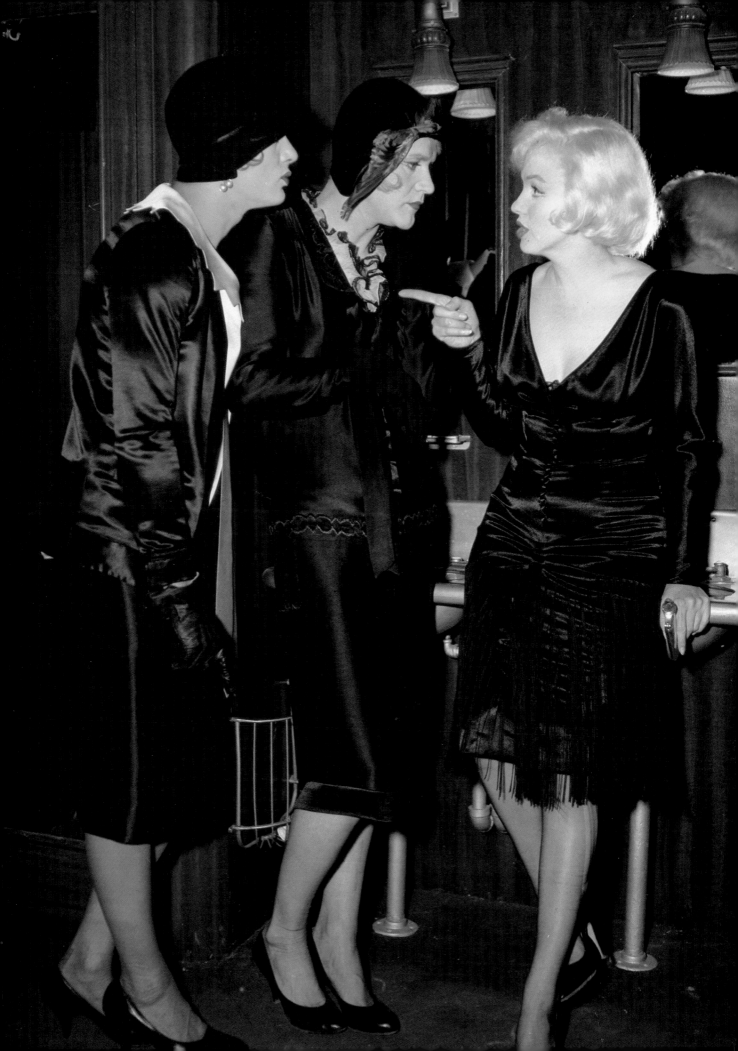

THE END OF THE AFFAIR

Let's Make Love cast Marilyn as a showgirl yet again, this time in a cabaret revue which satirizes a billionaire played by Yves Montand. He seeks her out, and by way of numerous convolutions, eventually they realize they are made for each other. According to Lena Pepitone that is just how it was in real life, after Simone Signoret was called back to Europe for filming. Certainly, whatever it was between them, director George Cukor commented that it made Marilyn more tractable and cooperative during the actual production. But such a relationship did not survive the end of shooting, for directly it was all over Montand packed his bags and returned to France – and Simone Signoret.

As a musical it was a film that just never managed to shake the lead from its feet; it lumbered. Although Marilyn sang such standards as 'My Heart Belongs to Daddy' the film's heart seemed to belong to some computer which had come up with this as the best way to please an audience. Many critics were displeased with the result. Justin Gilbert of the *New York Daily Mirror* said that Marilyn didn't have 'a single bright line', although another noted that the night he saw it the people he was with broke into applause. Marilyn herself could have done with that applause at the time. Her personal life she admitted was in a mess and she felt that she was not getting the movies that might at

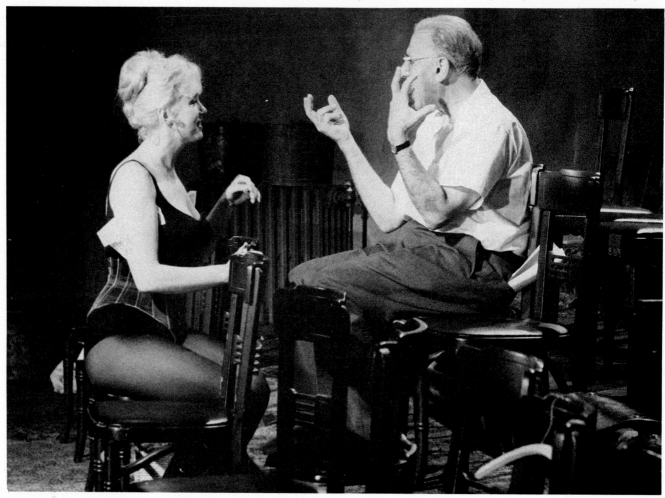

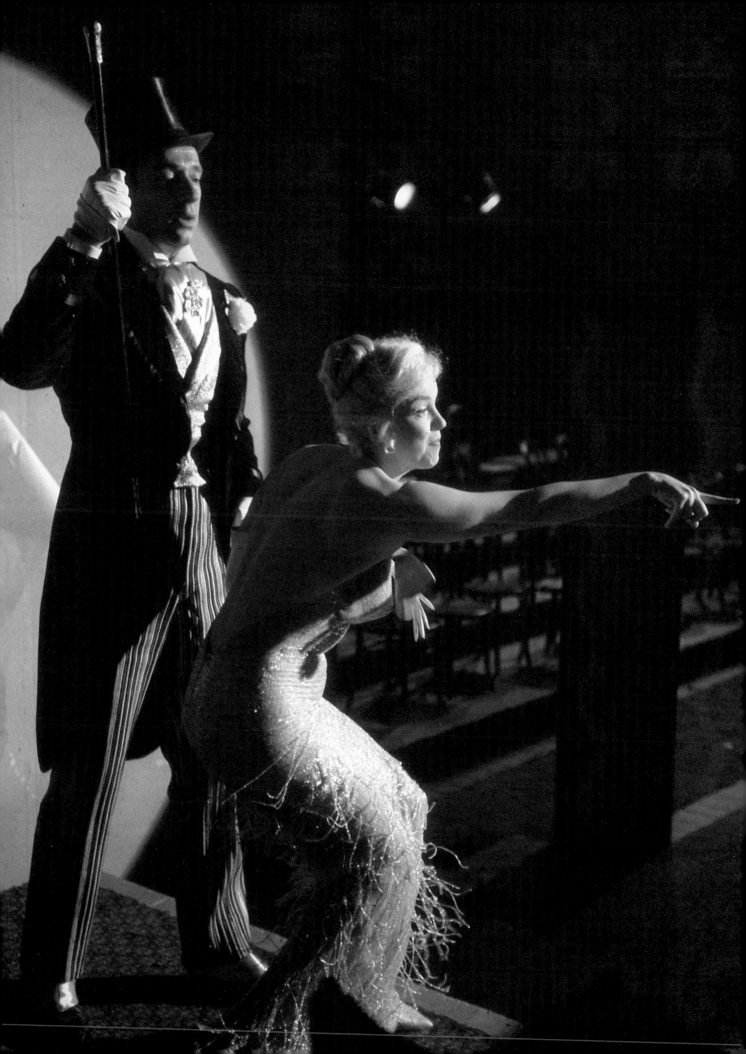

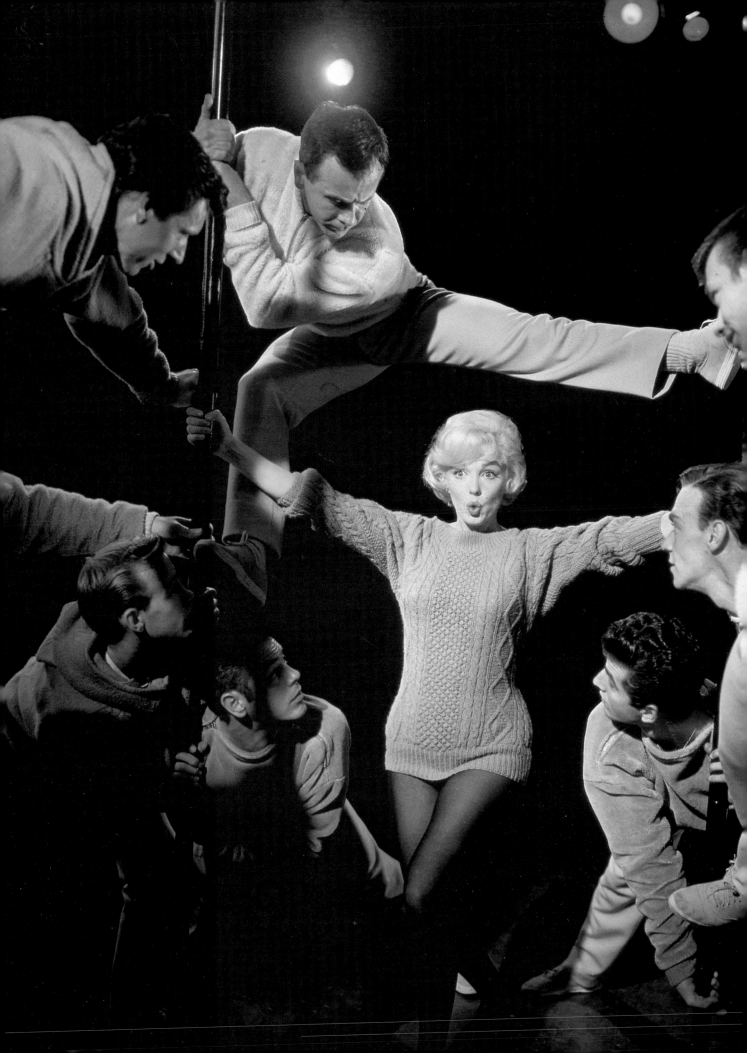

least show other professionals that she was up there with them in the major leagues. There was one hope, though, and that was in the film that Arthur Miller had written, which was called *The Misfits*.

The story concerns three ageing cowboys who drive wild horses out of the mountains near Reno, frightening them with planes, then rope them from a fast-moving truck and sell them for dog food. Marilyn's role: a divorcee who falls in love with the principal cowboy, yet is unable to understand what he does for a living. Miller's script shows the way the American pioneering spirit has been corrupted by commercialism.

Eli Wallach played one of the cowboys and Montgomery Clift another: he was a fine actor, of a self-destructive nature, of whom Marilyn said he was the only person she had met who was in worse shape than she was. She herself was in pretty bad shape, by now completely relying on tablets to get her up in the morning and to put her to sleep at night. Despite this she still suffered from acute insomnia. She promised, though, to try to be on time and not to cause any trouble on *The Misfits*, especially as her hero, Clark Gable, was playing the leading cowboy with whom she falls in love. Gable, 'The King', was already a legend when Marilyn was born; she remembered that she had fantasized that, in fact, he might have been her real father. Now, at 59, he was still a tough, charismatic figure, but, as he said, 'awful tired'.

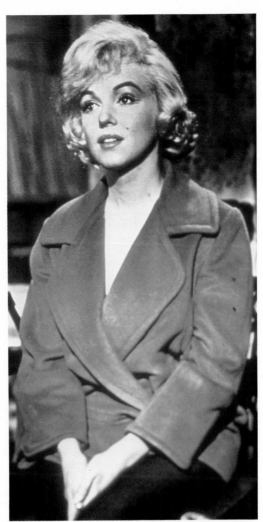

Left: A rather mannish coat for Marilyn in *Let's Make Love* (Twentieth Century-Fox), but anything less masculine than its effect cannot be imagined.

Left: Perhaps their troubled lives drew Marilyn and Montgomery Clift together. Seen here in *The Misfits* (United Artists), they had a good relationship off screen.

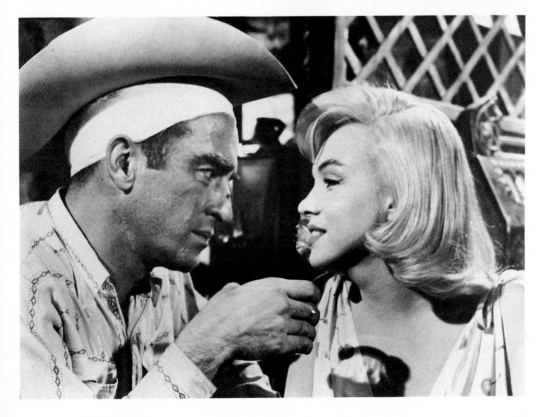

Far left: One of the production numbers from *Let's Make Love* (Twentieth Century-Fox) was 'My Heart Belongs to Daddy', Cole Porter's standard. Marilyn proves she looks as good in a man's sweater as in anything.

Clark Gable was the idol of young Norma Jean before she became Marilyn Monroe, and Marilyn was thrilled to work with him in *The Misfits* (United Artists) and hurt when it was suggested that troubles in the shooting might have accelerated his death.

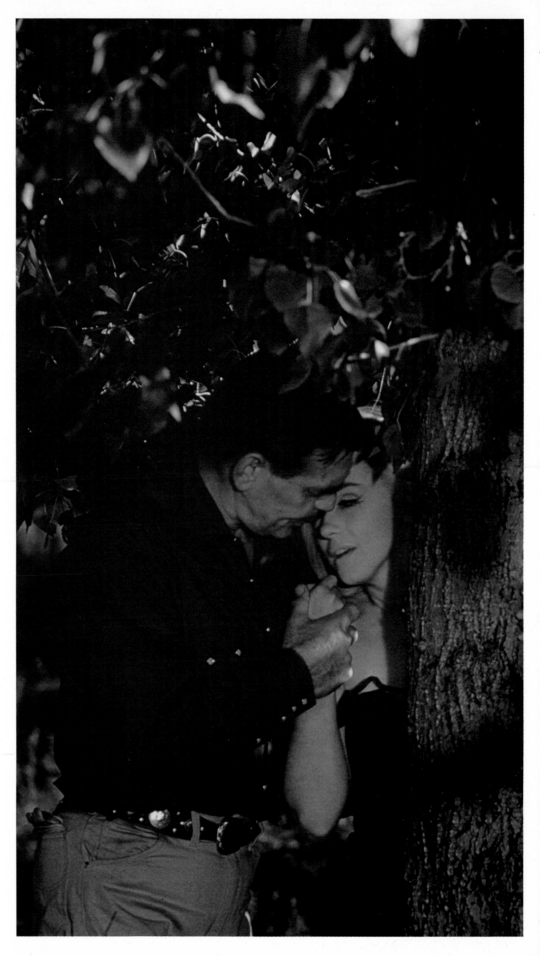

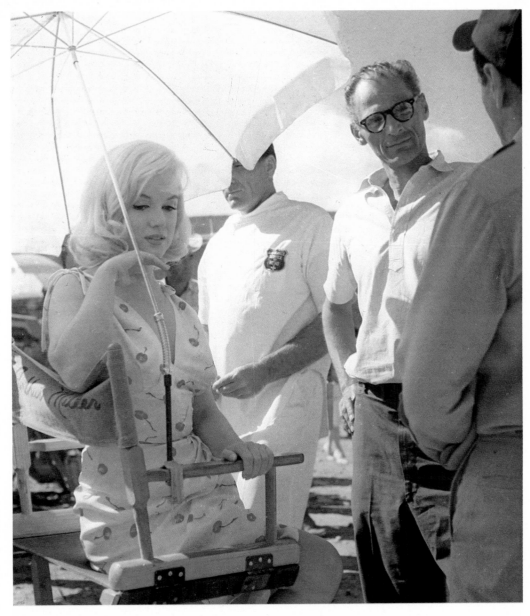

As scriptwriter, Marilyn's husband Arthur Miller was constantly on location for *The Misfits*, and indeed Marilyn is sitting in his chair, but she often ignored him, and their marriage was beginning to break up.

It was to be a nerve-wracking and gruelling film. Horses had to be ridden at breakneck speed – although stunt men were used closeups often called for the principals to do the riding – and Clark Gable had a bad back. And, despite her good resolutions, Marilyn was holding up the production with her lateness and illnesses which may well have been psychosomatic.

The director was John Huston, who had first worked with Marilyn on *The Asphalt Jungle* and knowing of Marilyn's reputation for being late on the set he had the daily call changed from 9.00 am to 10.00 am, to try to make things easier for her. It didn't. Clark Gable would drive out in his sports car, rehearse his lines then open a book. He never complained, no matter what time Marilyn showed up.

Although Marilyn seemed to be in a daze a lot of the time, she could also be wonderfully effective. It wasn't so much acting, Huston thought, as dragging something up from her subconscious, something which looked marvellous on screen.

Huston, though, was only too well aware that Arthur Miller and Marilyn were on the verge of breaking up. 'One evening I was about to drive away from the location – miles out in the desert – when I saw Arthur standing alone. Marilyn and her friends hadn't offered him a ride back; they'd just left him. If I hadn't happened to see him he would have been stranded out there. My sympathies were more and more with him.'

As a director, he was far too honest about her talent not to realize how remarkable she could be. 'I never felt Marilyn's much-publicized sexual attraction in the flesh, but on the screen it came across forcefully. But there was much more to her than that. She was appreciated as an artist in Europe long

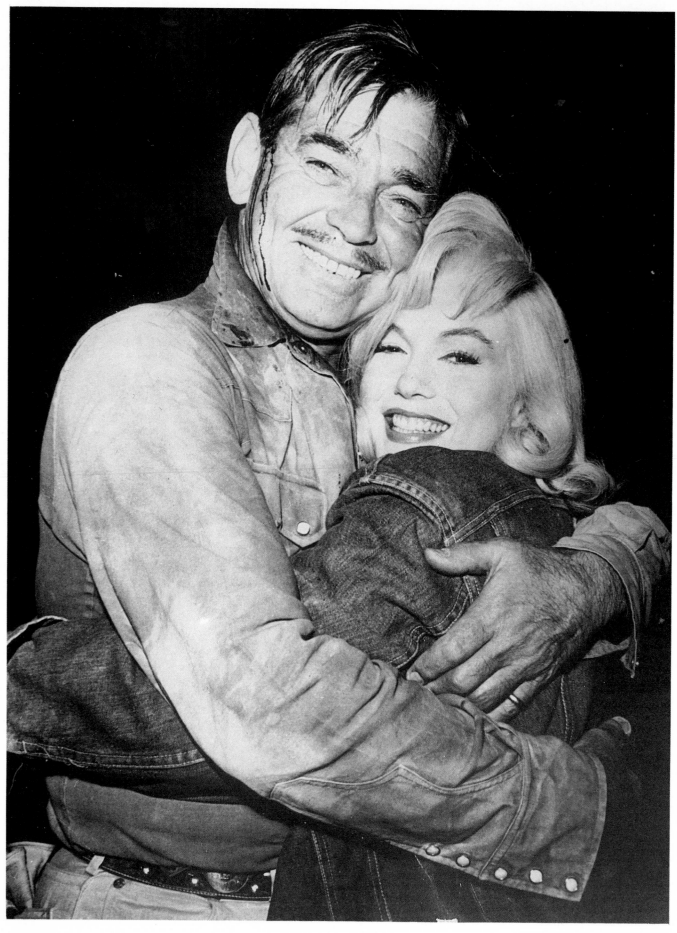

64

before her acceptance as anything but a sex symbol in the United States. Jean-Paul Sartre considered Marilyn Monroe the finest actress alive. He wanted her to play the leading female role in *Freud*.'

Marilyn was not so happy with herself, nor with *The Misfits*, which was around forty days over schedule and had been filmed in black and white ('you'd have thought they could afford colour'). The days after shooting finished were not happy for her either, as Clark Gable died in mid-November of a heart attack which some said had been brought on by the aggravation caused on *The Misfits*. The aftermath, therefore, seemed but a naturally gloomy extension to what had gone on during production. The reviews by the critics were, however, kinder than the circumstances surrounding the shooting. Said Paul V. Becker in the *New York Herald Tribune*: 'Here Miss Monroe is magic . . .

not a living pin-up dangled in skin tight satin before our eyes.' Another wrote: 'Hers is a dramatic, serious, accurate performance.' Balm for the wounds, but not balm enough. The marriage to Arthur Miller was now over. She felt that she had come away from the marriage with nothing; at least *he* had material for a play, *After the Fall*, which he was to write after her death.

It was, though, Twentieth Century-Fox insisted, time for work, under the contract by which she still owed them a film. *Something's Got to Give* was to be the title and its story was of a wife who returns from apparent death in a yacht accident to embarrass her husband (Dean Martin), who has made other plans for his life. Marilyn went to work with director George Cukor and one celebrated scene was shot in a swimming pool – that of Marilyn nude. It was to have been her 30th film.

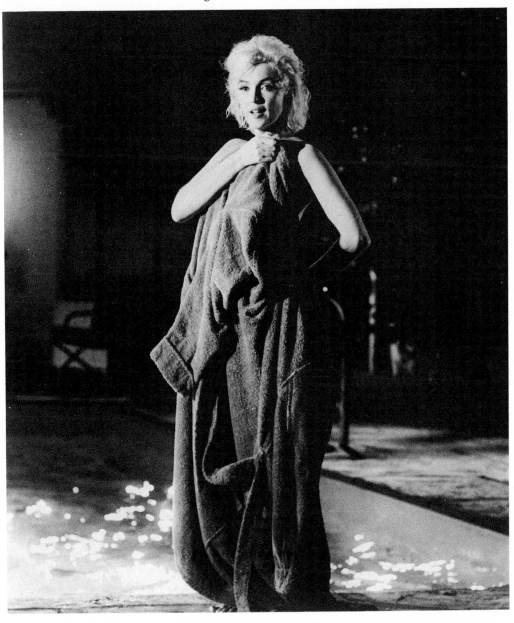

Left: In her last, unfinished, film, *Something's Got to Give* (Twentieth Century-Fox), Marilyn allowed herself to be photographed nude for the first time since the infamous calendar session many years before. Here she has just emerged from the swimming pool.

Far left: Marilyn and Clark Gable bidding farewell to each other after the last scenes shot of *The Misfits*. This happy occasion for Marilyn soon turned to sadness, as a few days later Gable suffered a fatal coronary attack.

Marilyn was never happy with the script and her old habits of lateness began to re-emerge. Production stopped, and was never to resume. Then Twentieth Century-Fox did what nobody had ever thought a studio would do in the circumstances, knowing Marilyn's deepening neurosis. The company filed suit against her 'for wilful violation of contract'. It was a bitter blow. Marilyn went into deep seclusion and could only be reached by close personal friends such as the Strasbergs, who put it about that Marilyn was contemplating the stage and a role in 'Anna Christie'. Joe DiMaggio, with whom she had continued to be friendly after their divorce, was always on hand. And, of course, there were doctors. There were always doctors.

But on 5 August 1962, there was nobody around when Marilyn most needed them. There was evidence that she had tried to phone people, leaving her telephone number on doctors' answering machines. On a chair were some legal documents that she seems to have been reading; documents concerning her legal wrangle with Twentieth Century-Fox. But there were also, on the table beside her bed, bottles of pills. And Marilyn Monroe was dead.

The housekeeper, awakened by 'an uneasy feeling', found her at three o'clock in the morning. All over the world millions of people who had regarded Marilyn Monroe as standing for something bright and vital and part of their own lives found themselves in a state of shock. The coroner's report said that it was 'probable suicide'; certainly her dying was the result of an overdose of barbiturates. But those who take such pills know how easy it is to take too many; the mind cannot remember the count of how many have been swallowed.

All the judgements simply meant that a light had been snuffed out. The light that was Marilyn Monroe. And in Los Angeles Jim Dougherty said to his second wife: 'Say a prayer for Norma Jean. She's dead.'

Even after their divorce, Marilyn continued to have a strong affection for Joe DiMaggio, and often liked to be with him, particularly at low moments.

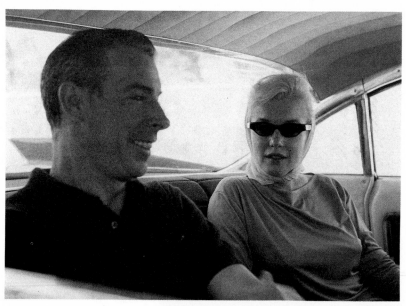

Right: Marilyn's funeral casket, covered with flowers, being taken from the chapel to the cemetery. The pallbearers are Alan Snyder, her make-up man, Sidney Guillsroff, her hairdresser, and four mortuary employees.

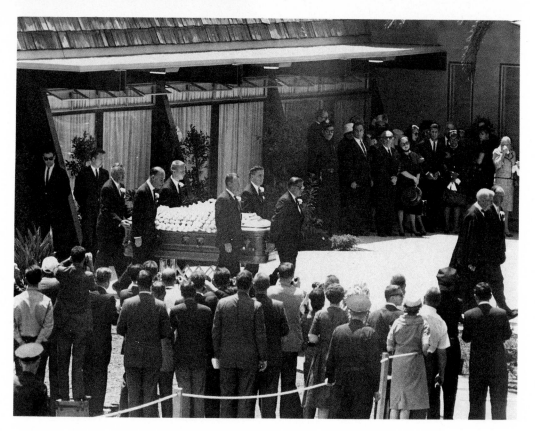

EPILOGUE

Marilyn Monroe was 36 when she died and *Something's Got to Give* would have been her 30th film. It was an ironical title considering what happened to her, and an irony at which she might well have giggled. It still seems incredible and unbelievable, remembering her on-screen personality, to believe that she is really gone from the cinema and the world. In his funeral address Lee Strasberg said of her: 'The dream of her talent, which she had nurtured as a child, was not a mirage. When she first came to me I was amazed at the sterling sensitivity which she possessed and which had remained fresh and undimmed, struggling to express itself despite the life to which she had been subjected.'

There was obviously something more than just physical beauty in her, something in her performances with which people identified. She had 'a luminous quality – a combination of wistfulness, radiance, yearning – to set her apart and yet make everyone wish to be part of it, to share in the child-like naiveté which was at once so shy and yet so vibrant . . .' She was a sensitive artist and woman who brought joy and pleasure to the world.

Joy and pleasure, of course, but, to a certain extent, after her death – guilt. As Fred Lawrence Guiles wrote: 'None of Marilyn's

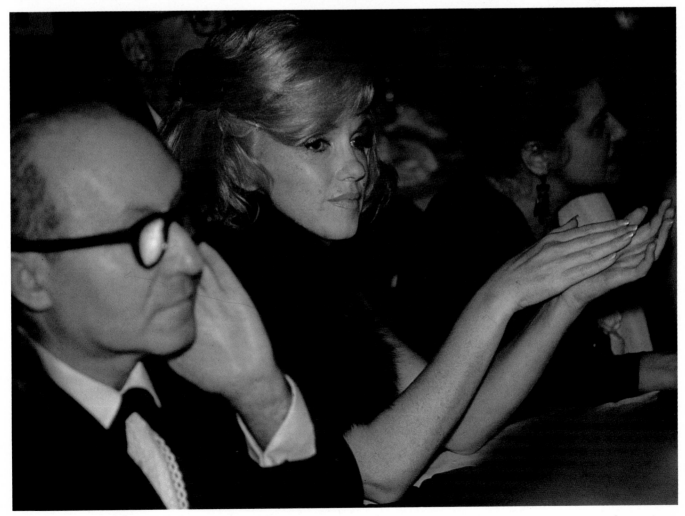

Marilyn as guest of honour at an Actors Studio benefit party, sitting between her old friends Lee and Paula Strasberg.

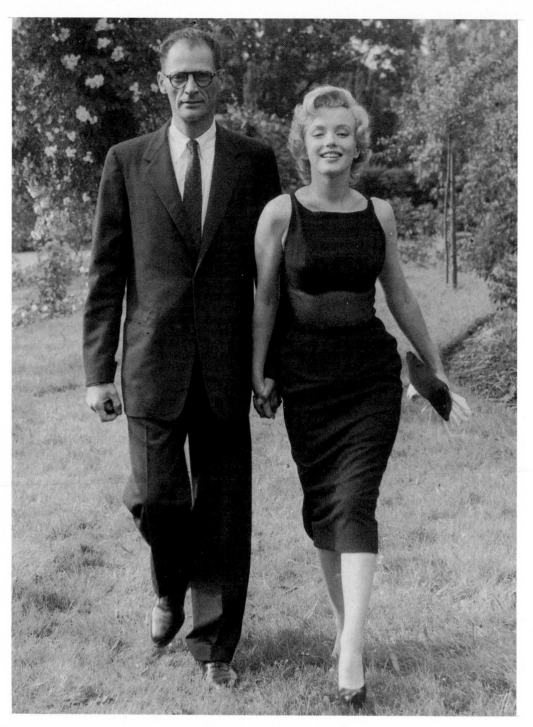

Marilyn with her third husband Arthur Miller. She was a great reader, and it was once suggested, not wholly in jest, that her brains and his beauty made a good match.

friends, husbands and lovers escaped a profound sense of guilt that was to supersede for a time, and in some instances for all time, the warm memory of a young woman with laughter ready at her lips, a laughter sometimes wry perhaps, but none the less there.'

Yet the self-destructive pattern of her life made her early death seem inevitable.

Arthur Miller himself tried to erase Marilyn's memory from his own life with a play, *After the Fall*, in which the childlike actress Maggie is not unlike Marilyn. He regarded it, he said, as no more autobiographical than his other plays, but the critics were unani-mous in seeing that Maggie and Marilyn were one and the same.

There were all kinds of theories regarding her death; that the Kennedys, John F. and Bobby, were somehow involved. But as Lena Pepitone was to write: 'It was, and has been, frequently whispered that Marilyn was having an affair with President Kennedy, or his brother Bobby, or both. Marilyn didn't get mad at these rumours, though. She just laughed. The Kennedys, whom she had met through Frank Sinatra's friend Peter Law-ford (then the husband of a Kennedy sister, Pat), were "cute", Marilyn said. She liked them because they were funny and smart. "But they're not my type. They're boys." '

But, in a more general aspect, many who never met her in person felt that guilt; her audiences, even. As though somehow they had betrayed her. It was something she was aware of when I met her on a couple of occasions: this sense of treachery for some unspecified crime. She had been reading Kafka's 'The Trial' in which the hero Josef K. is arrested for a criminal act which is never described and of which he is not aware.

She was always a great reader, as if trying to catch up with her lack of real education, to fill in those gaping holes of which she was too much aware. Her comments on 'The Trial' when I met her at Egham were perceptive. 'It's like we all feel, this sense of guilt. I know they say it's the Jewish thing with Kafka – that's what Arthur (Miller) says anyway – but it goes beyond that. It's about all men and women. This sense that we have fallen or something. I suppose that's what they mean by Original Sin.' It was a strange conversation to be having with a supposed sex-symbol, but our interview was a strange one, anyway. People drifted in and out, not being introduced; the first time I met her was in the morning when she seemed tired and disorientated. The second was late afternoon when she seemed more composed and relaxed.

One of the matters which exercised her very much were the critics' reactions to her. She didn't need them, she said vehemently, but judging by the way she constantly returned to the subject she felt that they ought to need her. She admitted to a preference for Bosley Crowther, but that was all; the rest were just writing 'to make headlines'. But looking through 'The Films of Marilyn Monroe' edited by Michael Conway and Mark Ricci, the quotes of favour come early, surprisingly early, in her career. In her way Marilyn was always to some extent the Critics' Choice.

Even as far back as *Ladies of the Chorus* Tibor Krekes in the *Motion Picture Herald* was writing about it: 'One of the bright spots is Miss Monroe's singing. She is pretty and, with her pleasing voice and style, she shows promise.' Her prowess in *Love Happy* rated no comment at all, but possibly because everyone was too besotted with the Marx Brothers and their looney antics. *The Asphalt Jungle*, though, unleashed a few superlatives for Marilyn amid all the comments on the film itself. Liza Wilson wrote in *Photoplay*: 'This picture is packed with standout performances . . . There's a beautiful blonde, too, name of Marilyn Monroe, who plays Calhern's girl friend and makes the most of her footage.'

Mostly, for some time after that, the comments from critics were about the movies themselves, not specifically Marilyn. *Let's Make It Legal*, though, had Frank Quinn, of the *New York Daily Mirror* saying: 'Marilyn Monroe parades her shapely chassis for incidental excitement.' And Wanda Hale in the *New York Daily News* wrote of Claudette Colbert and Macdonald Carey: 'Their presences and a satisfactory amount of bright dialogue counteract strained farcical situations and the indifferent story . . . Marilyn Monroe is amusing in a brief role as a beautiful shapely blonde who has her eye on Zachary Scott and his millions.'

Perhaps the most eulogistic comment came from Alton Cook in the *New York Telegram and Sun* about her role in *Clash by Night*: 'Perhaps we should mention the first full-length glimpse the picture gives us of Marilyn Monroe as an actress. The verdict is gratifyingly good. This girl has a refreshing exuberance, an abundance of girlish high spirits. She is a forceful actress, too, when crisis comes along. She has definitely stamped herself as a gifted new star, worthy

Marilyn had only a brief role in *Let's Make It Legal*, but her name appeared on the advertising posters. She received good notices from New York papers, who found her exciting and amusing.

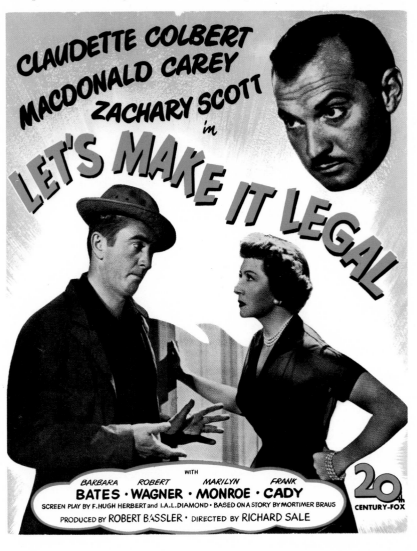

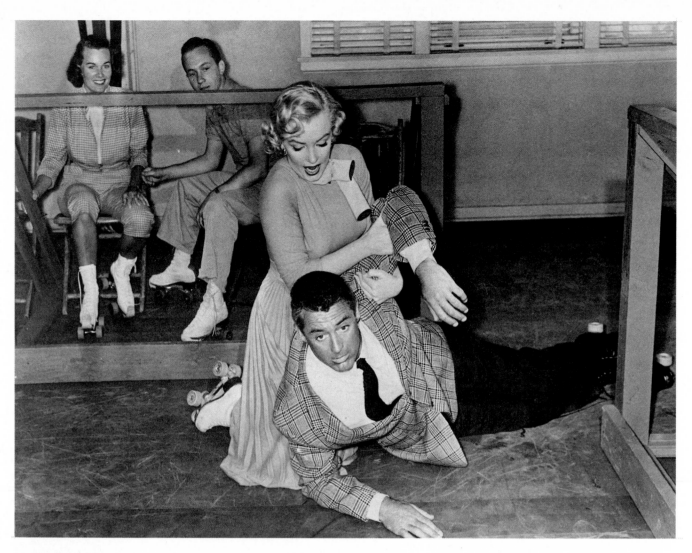

Marilyn thought the critics did not take her seriously in the dumb-blonde parts she played in a string of films in the early 1950s, including *Monkey Business* (Twentieth Century-Fox) with Cary Grant.

of all that fantastic press agentry. Her role here is not very big, but she makes it dominant.' Alton Cook, again, about *We're Not Married* wrote: 'Marilyn Monroe supplies the beauty at which she is Hollywood's currently foremost expert . . .'

John Huston told me about Marilyn: 'You know Hollywood is a great place for type-casting you – off screen as well as on. Because Marilyn was a blonde she was seen as a certain kind of girl. A gold-digger? Well, maybe that is the description. But I wouldn't put it like that, you see. After all I knew her when she was with Johnny Hyde and she was really very, very fond of him. If she'd wanted she could have married him and been a very rich widow. But I don't think she ever thought like that. She didn't calculate. That's why what she did went against that kind of type-casting. But there was this period when in all her films, including mine to a certain extent, she was portrayed and, in fact, did portray gold-diggers.'

Don't Bother to Knock, however, was the first film which saw her out of that typecast context. Bosley Crowther, in the *New York*

Times, was not impressed by her performance as a mentally disturbed baby-sitter, but Frank Quinn in the *New York Daily Mirror* thought 'she has good dramatic promise'.

He went on: 'She is what the movies need, a few more like her and the industry would thrive. Miss Monroe's delineation of the deranged beauty is a surprise. *Don't Bother to Knock* has good pace, an intriguing story and many assets – of which Marilyn Monroe is the most important.' Such a lift-off, though, got its own put-down with *Monkey Business* which was back to the dumb-blonde stakes again: 'Ginger Rogers and Cary Grant are assisted in this amusing nonsense by Marilyn Monroe who can look and act dumber than any of the screen's current blondes.'

'They never took me seriously in those days,' said Marilyn. 'There was no consistency in the way my career was handled by Fox. Up one minute, down the other. Dizzy blonde one minute, murderous adulterous the next.'

Strangely, she herself reckoned that the real watershed in her career came with *Niagara*, in which she played a seductress of

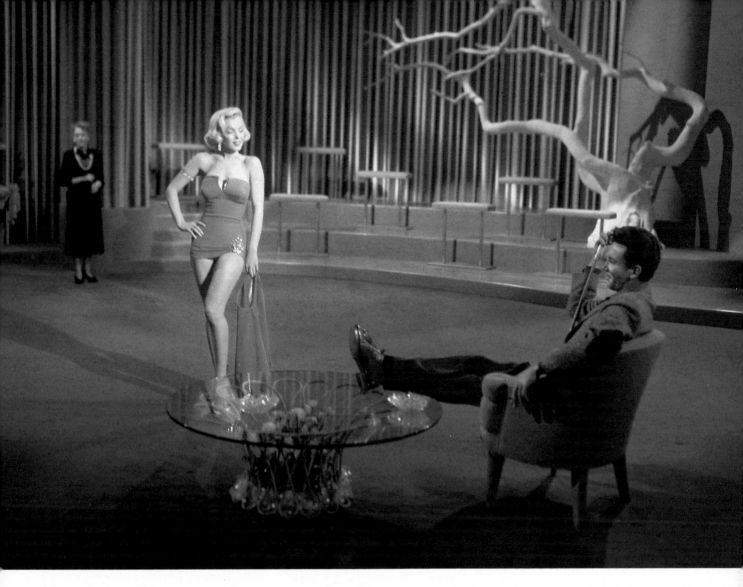

very few scruples. 'I felt I was having some control over my life and career,' she said. Certainly, the critics reeled over her special impact in this movie. Wrote Otis L. Guernsey Jr in the *New York Herald Tribune*: 'Miss Monroe plays the kind of wife whose dress, in the words of the script "is cut so low you can see her knees". The dress is red; the actress has very nice knees and, under Henry Hathaway's direction she gives the kind of serpentine performance that makes the audience hate her while admiring her, which is proper for the story.' Wrote A. H. Weiler in the *New York Times*: 'Perhaps Miss Monroe is not the perfect actress at this point. But neither the director nor the gentlemen who handled the cameras appeared to be concerned with this. They have caught every possible curve both in the intimacy of the boudoir and in equally revealing tight dresses. And they have illustrated pretty concretely that she can be seductive – even when she walks.'

Pitted against other glamour queens – Betty Grable and Lauren Bacall – in *How to Marry a Millionaire* she proved that she

could still hold her own in the art of projecting. Said Otis L. Guernsey: 'Her magnificent proportions are as appealing as ever, and her stint as a deadpan comedienne is as nifty as her looks. Playing a near-sighted charmer who won't wear her glasses when men are around she bumps into the furniture and reads books upside down with a limpid guile that nearly melts the screen.'

Even more serious aspects of Marilyn, as in *River of No Return*, brought comments about the way she looked. Wrote Bosley Crowther in the *New York Times:* 'It is a toss-up whether the scenery or the adornment of Marilyn Monroe is the feature of greater attraction in *River of No Return* . . . The mountainous scenery is spectacular but so, in her own way, is Miss Monroe. The patron's preference, if any, probably will depend upon which he's interested in.'

'Always the way I looked, never what I could do,' she was later to complain. But there was an affection in such critical comments which showed that she had become a national symbol, an institution, a sexual mascot to be regarded rather endearingly. And

In *How to Marry a Millionaire* (Twentieth Century-Fox) Marilyn had competition in both acting and beauty from Betty Grable and Lauren Bacall, but critics agreed that she easily held her own.

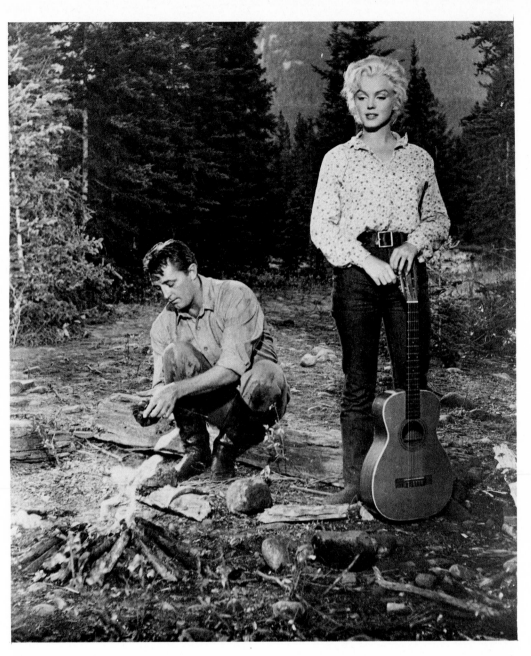

Critic Bosley Crowther wrote of *River of No Return* (Twentieth Century-Fox) that 'it is a toss-up whether the scenery or the adornment of Marilyn Monroe is the feature of greater attraction'.

when films such as *The Seven Year Itch* cashed in on that particular projection of attraction then the comment was apt and due, as in this from Philip Strasberg of the *New York Daily Mirror*: 'Her pouting delivery, puckered lips – the personification of this decade's glamour – make her one of Hollywood's top attractions, which she again proves here as the not too bright model.'

The way she looked . . . even in a serious movie such as *Bus Stop* it was the surface appearance that the critics looked at first – and were promptly amazed. Said Bosley Crowther in the *New York Times*: 'The striking fact is that Josh Logan has got her to do a great deal more than wiggle and pout and pop her big eyes and play the synthetic vamp in this film. He has got her to be the beat-up B-girl of Mr Inge's play, even down

to the Ozark accent and the look of pellagra about the skin. He has got her to be the tinselled floozie, the semi-moronic doll who is found in a Phoenix clip-joint by a cowboy of equally limited brains and is hotly pursued by this suitor to a snow-bound bus stop in the Arizona wilds. And what's most important he has got her to light the small flame of dignity that splutters pathetically in this chippie and to make a rather moving sort of her.'

One of the qualities of Marilyn was her ability, perhaps unwitting, to invest what she did with a quality that transcended the merely physical. Her looks and manner had a sly innocence, a seductive naiveté: she was just made to be rescued by a knight on a white charger. Archer Winsten in the *New York Post* once described Marilyn as 'half-

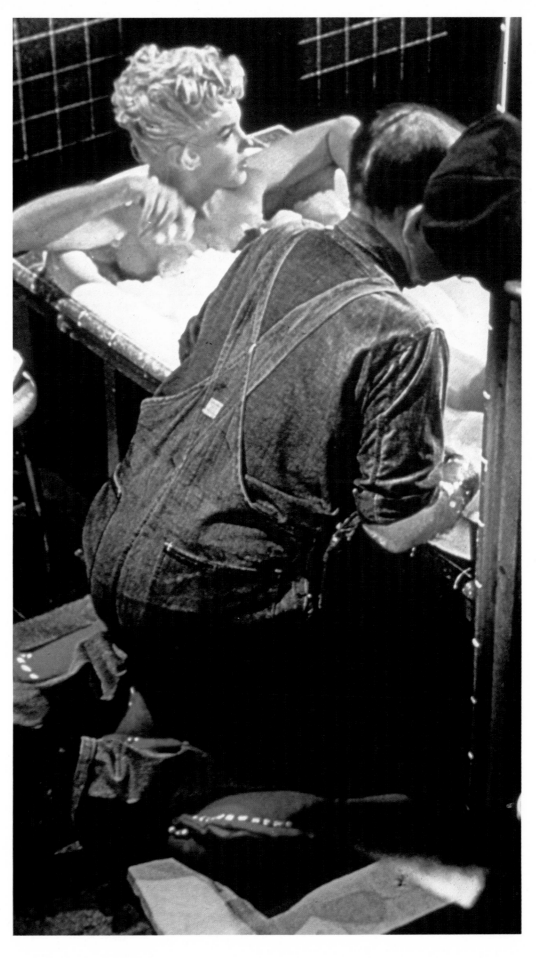

Marilyn sometimes complained that critics were over-keen on the way she looked, but as she played scenes like this in *The Seven Year Itch* (Twentieth Century-Fox), in which her toe was caught in the bath tap, it was hardly surprising.

73

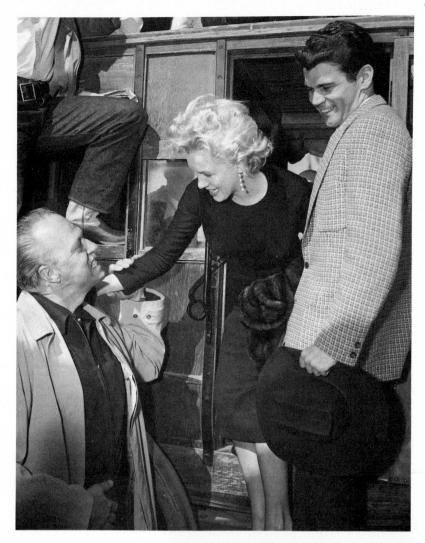

sensation' – a description meant to convey that what she had was a mixture of sensitivity and sensibility of a kind.

Frankie Vaughan, the British singer, who worked on *Let's Make Love*, was very much aware, he says, that she was the star of that film. 'And she deserved to be. But it was interesting to watch. When I worked with her she always seemed to be on time for shooting, none of those notorious late starts. And when she came on everybody sort of smartened up. It was as though the very fact of her presence was the light that fell on everyone and we were all aware that the star had arrived. Certainly, she seemed to me to be very professional in all she did.'

Lena Pepitone wrote that this professional romanticism also extended into her private life: 'She talked about the Fred Astaire movies of her youth – top hat, white tie and tails, dressing up, champagne, caviar – and not all alone in her room. She wanted to do the town: "Isn't that what New York's all about? I just need the right guy to do it with." Perhaps Yves Montand was the closest Marilyn ever came to this dream of sophistication. He was debonair, European, charming, but she never mentioned him any more. Marilyn knew how to forget certain deep hurts. It was one important way she was able to survive.'

Arthur Miller, too, perceived the 'deep hurts' when he said of her: 'Marilyn identifies powerfully with all living things, but her extraordinary embrace of life is intermingled with great sadness.' He it was, too, who saw

Above: Josh Logan, seen here greeting Marilyn and co-star Don Murray, obtained from Marilyn an acting performance which some think her best, when he directed her in *Bus Stop*.

Right: Yves Montand perhaps came closest to one ideal of Marilyn's – a sophisticated man who could escort her around New York. They met on the set of *Let's Make Love*.

Far right: Frankie Vaughan with Marilyn in a scene from *Let's Make Love* (Twentieth Century-Fox). His view of her at work differed from the standard one. He found her very professional.

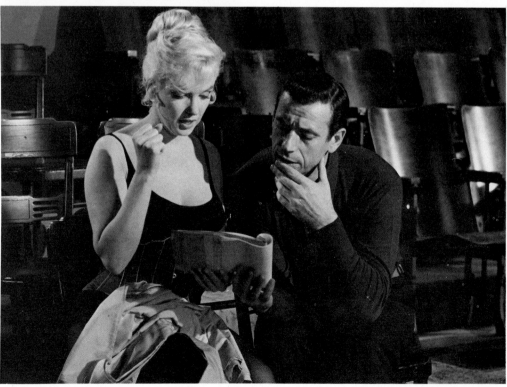

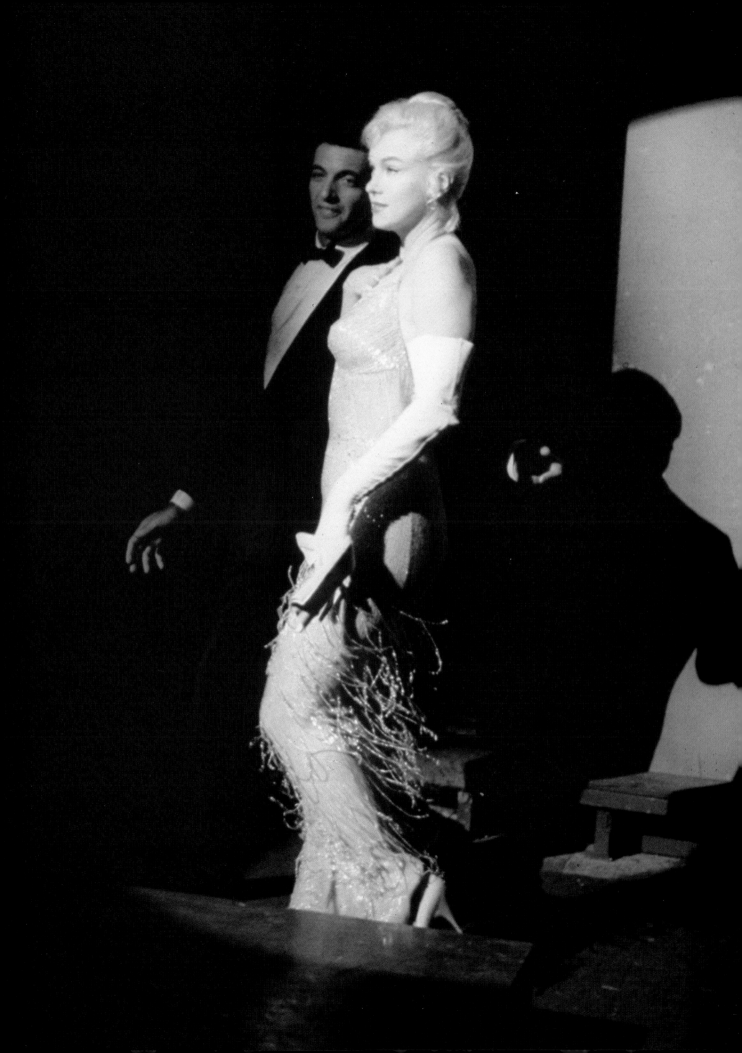

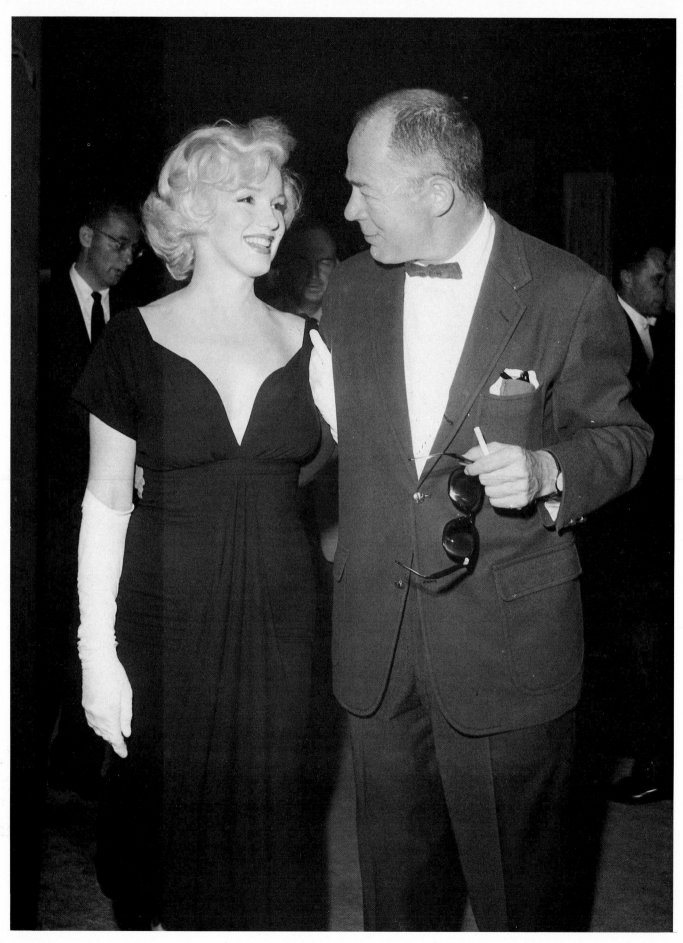

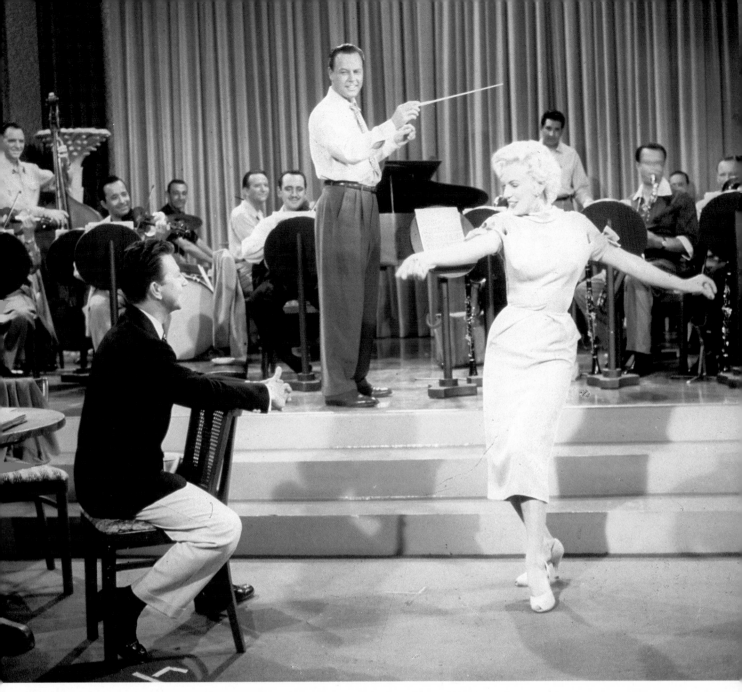

how serious she was about her acting: 'In a whole picture there may be only two scenes of which she is really proud. She has great respect for the ideal of acting, so great that some part of her is always put to shame by the distance between what she achieves and the goal that she has set herself.'

Marilyn, in fact, took herself seriously because everybody else did. Even when they were disparaging of her talents that meant that they accepted her as a fact of their lives. Said Billy Wilder: 'God gave her everything. The first day a photographer took a picture of her she was a genius.' He later said he regretted having said it. 'When you've worked with her, though, there's a chance that you see her very differently from the way outsiders do.'

Perhaps it was those outsiders who knew

her best of all. The British poetess, Dame Edith Sitwell, met Marilyn while she was in Hollywood – a strange meeting, indeed! – and described her later as looking like 'a beautiful ghost. A visitor from some other plane; only here visiting.'

In that funeral eulogy, Lee Strasberg also said: 'In her own lifetime she created a myth of what a poor girl from a deprived background could attain. For the entire world she became a symbol of the eternal feminine . . .

'This quality was even more evident when she was on stage. I am truly sorry that the public who loved her did not have the opportunity to see her as we did, in many of the roles that foreshadowed what she would have become. Without a doubt she would have been one of the really great actresses of the stage.'

Above: Marilyn in *There's No Business like Show Business* (Twentieth Century-Fox). She epitomized one show-business canon herself – that a poor girl can get to the top.

Left: Billy Wilder, with a radiant Marilyn at a press conference for the film *Some Like It Hot*, said of her: 'God gave her everything.' He had less flattering views about working with her, however.

Eulogies, farewells, testaments to a star fallen from the heavens of an audience's adulation: like candles, such mythic personalities are blown out in the wind of too much, too soon. Of the times I met Marilyn nothing vital really extrudes from a mass of words; only impressions. A 'beautiful ghost' is an apt and rare summing up of how you felt when with her, as people – her courtiers – drifted in and out, inserting comments, letting her know that they were around and on her register of paid employees.

When I left her I remember that she looked up at me, her eyes slightly blurred, perhaps from the tablets we were later told she was on – there was no instance of it that I noticed – and said apropos of nothing: 'Too many people. Too many people.'

It was as good an exit line as any. And a better farewell than most. Perhaps it was what she said just before she died. It would have been entirely appropriate.

Of course, it is not the end. We can go on seeing her. That is our privilege and our pleasure. Marilyn Monroe, born Norma Jean, paid our dues for us on those accounts. For she was a woman who all her life had been living on the edge of the volcano, only to fall over that edge at the end. That she managed to climb up there though, in the first place, says something about her – and the human spirit.

Right: Décolleté triumphant. Marilyn as she will probably be best remembered. In a Miss America Pageant Ride of 1952 she exuded vitality.

Far right: Marilyn in sunny and more reflective mood off-set for *The Misfits*. This was the last film she was to complete.

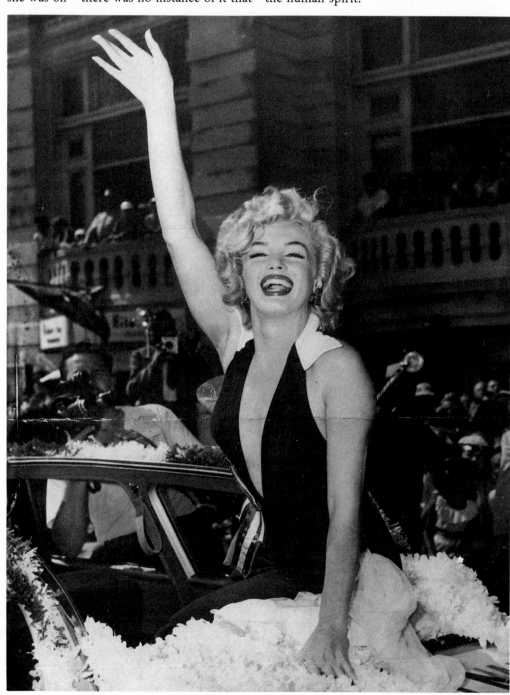

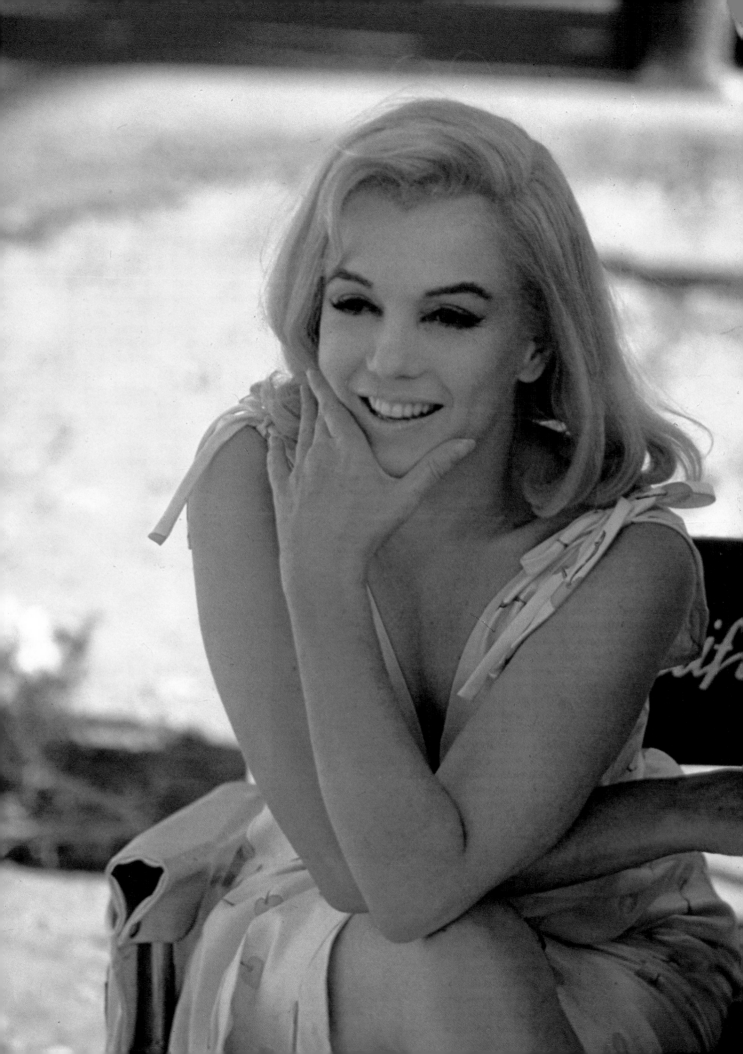

FILMOGRAPHY

Scudda Hoo! Scudda Hay! (later changed to *Summer Lightning*).   1948. Twentieth Century-Fox. Director: F. Hugh Herbert. With June Haver, Lon McCallister.

Dangerous Years.   1947. Twentieth Century-Fox. Director: Arthur Pierson. With William Halop, Ann E. Todd, Scotty Beckett, Jerome Cowan.

Ladies of the Chorus.   1949. Columbia. Director: Phil Karlson. With Adele Jergens, Rand Brooks, Nana Bryant.

Love Happy.   1949. United Artists. Director: David Miller. With the Marx Brothers, Ilona Massey, Vera-Ellen.

A Ticket to Tomahawk.   1950. Twentieth Century-Fox. Director: Richard Sale. With Dan Dailey, Anne Baxter, Rory Calhoun, Walter Brennan.

The Asphalt Jungle.   1950. Metro-Goldwyn-Mayer. Director: John Huston. With Sterling Hayden, Louish Calhern, Jean Hagen, James Whitmore, Sam Jaffe.

The Fireball.   1950. Twentieth Century-Fox. Director: Tay Garnett. With Mickey Rooney, Pat O'Brien.

All About Eve.   1950. Twentieth Century-Fox. Director: Joseph L. Mankiewicz. With Bette Davis, Anne Baxter, George Sanders.

Right Cross.   1950. Metro-Goldwyn-Mayer. Director: John Sturges. With June Allyson, Dick Powell, Ricardo Montalban.

Home Town Story.   1951. Metro-Goldwyn-Mayer. Director: Arthur Pierson. With Jeffrey Lynn, Donald Crisp.

As Young as You Feel.   1951. Twentieth Century-Fox. Director: Harmon Jones. With Monty Woolley, Thelma Ritter, David Wayne.

Love Nest.   1951. Twentieth Century-Fox. Director: Joseph Newman. With June Haver, William Lundigan, Frank Fay.

Let's Make It Legal.   1951. Twentieth Century-Fox. Director: Richard Sale. With Claudette Colbert, Macdonald Carey, Zachary Scott.

Clash by Night.   1952. RKO Radio-Jerry Wald and Norman Krasna Productions. Director: Fritz Lang. With Barbara Stanwyck, Paul Douglas, Robert Ryan.

We're Not Married.   1952. Twentieth Century-Fox. Director: Edmund Goulding. With Ginger Rogers, Fred Allen, Victor Moore.

Don't Bother to Knock.   1952. Twentieth Century-Fox. Director: Roy Ward Baker. With Richard Widmark, Anne Bancroft.

Monkey Business.   1952. Twentieth Century-Fox. Director: Howard Hawks. With Cary Grant, Ginger Rogers, Charles Coburn.

O.Henry's Full House.   1952. Twentieth Century-Fox. Director: Henry Koster. With Charles Laughton, David Wayne.

Niagara.   1953. Twentieth Century-Fox. Director: Henry Hathaway. With Joseph Cotten, Jean Peters, Casey Adams.

Gentlemen Prefer Blondes.   1953. Twentieth Century-Fox. Director: Howard Hawks. With Jane Russell, Charles Coburn.

How to Marry a Millionaire.   1953. Twentieth Century-Fox. Director: Jean Negulesco. With Betty Grable, Lauren Bacall, William Powell, David Wayne.

River of No Return.   1954. Twentieth Century-Fox. Director: Otto Preminger. With Robert Mitchum, Rory Calhoun.

There's No Business like Show Business.   1954. Twentieth Century-Fox. Director: Walter Lang. With Ethel Merman, Donald O'Connor, Dan Dailey.

The Seven Year Itch.   1955. Twentieth Century-Fox. Director: Billy Wilder. With Tom Ewell.

Bus Stop.   1956. Twentieth Century-Fox. Director: Joshua Logan. With Don Murray, Arthur O'Connell.

The Prince and the Showgirl.   1957. Warner Brothers – Marilyn Monroe Productions. Director: Laurence Olivier. With Laurence Olivier, Sybil Thorndike, Richard Wattis, Jeremy Spencer.

Some Like It Hot.   1959. United Artists. Director: Billy Wilder. With Tony Curtis, Jack Lemmon.

Let's Make Love.   1960. Twentieth Century-Fox. Director: George Cukor. With Yves Montand, Tony Randall, Frankie Vaughan.

The Misfits.   1961. United Artists. Director: John Huston. With Clark Gable, Montgomery Clift, Thelma Ritter, Eli Wallach.

Something's Got to Give.   1962. (Unfinished). Twentieth Century-Fox. Director: George Cukor. With Dean Martin, Cyd Charisse.